Advances in Transfusion Safety

Developments in Biologicals

Vol. 120

This series «Developments in Biologicals» begins with Vol. 102 and is the continuation of IABs symposia series «Progress in Immunobiological Standardization», Vols 1-5, «Immunobiological Standardization», Vols 1-22 and «Developments in Biological Standardization», Vols 23-101.

Organized and published by the International Association for Biologicals (IABs)

KARGER

Basel · Freiburg · Paris · London · New York ·
Bangalore · Bangkok · Singapore · Tokyo · Sydney

Advances in Transfusion Safety

Natcher Auditorium, National Institutes of Health (NIH) Bethesda, MD, USA, June 4-6, 2003

Volume editors

G.N. Vyas
University of San Francisco, San Francisco, California, USA

A.E. Williams
Food and Drug Administration, Rockville, Maryland, USA

Proceedings of a Symposium co-sponsored by:
U.S. Food and Drug Administration
AABB (formerly known as the American Association of Blood Banks)
National Heart, Lung, and Blood Institute, NIH
U.S. Department of Defense
International Association for Biologicals (IABs)

26 figures and 33 tables, 2005

KARGER

Basel · Freiburg · Paris · London · New York ·
Bangalore · Bangkok · Singapore · Tokyo · Sydney

• • • • • • • • • • • • • • • • •

Developments in Biologicals

Library of Congress Cataloging-in-Publication Data

Advances in transfusion safety: Natcher Auditorium, National Institutes of Health (NIH), Bethesda, MD, USA, June 4-6, 2003 / volume editors, G.N. Vyas, A.E. Williams; proceedings of a symposium co-sponsored by U.S. Food and Drug Administration... [et al.].
p. ; cm. -- (Developments in biologicals ; v. 120)
Includes bibliographical references.
ISBN 3-8055-7935-7 (soft cover: alk. paper)
1. Blood--Transfusion--Safety measures--Congresses. 2. Blood--Collection and preservation--Safety measures--Congresses.
[DNLM: 1. Blood Banks--standards--Congresses. 2. Blood Transfusion--standards--Congresses. 3. Blood Donors Congresses. 4. Disease--Transmission--prevention & control--Congresses. 5. Safety standards Congresses. WH 460 A2444 2005] I. Vyas, Girish N. II. Williams, A. E. (Alan E.), 1950- III. United States. Food and Drug Administration. IV. Series.
RM171.3.A38 2005
362.17'84--dc22 2005014652

Bibliographic Indices. This publication is listed in bibliographic services, including Current Contents® and Index Medicus.

Drug dosage. The authors and the publisher have exerted every effort to ensure that drug selection and dosage set forth in this text are in accord with current recommendations and practice at the time of publication. However, in view of ongoing research, changes in government regulations, and the constant flow of information relating to drug therapy and drug reactions, the reader is urged to check the package insert for each drug for any change in indications and dosage and for added warnings and precautions. This is particularly important when the recommended agent is a new and/or infrequently employed drug.

Printed in Switzerland by Médecine et Hygiène, Genève.
ISBN 3-8055-7935-7

Scientific Program Committee

J.S. Epstein	Co-chair, Rockville, MD, USA
R.Y. Dodd	Co-chair, Rockville, MD, USA
J.P. Allain	Cambridge, UK
H.J. Alter	Bethesda, MD, USA
B.M. Alving	Bethesda, MD, USA
H.G. Klein	Bethesda, MD, USA
R.M. Lewis	Rockville, MD, USA
J.S. Robertson	Potters Bar, UK
R. Seitz	Langen, Germany
C. Smit Sibinga	Groningen, the Netherlands
P.F. Strengers	Amsterdam, the Netherlands
G.N. Vyas	San Francisco, CA, USA
A.E. Williams	Rockville, MD, USA

Organisation of the Scientific Program

Session I	Current Status of Blood Safety Moderator: *J.S. Epstein*
Session II	New Safety Technologies I Moderator: *H.J. Alter*
Session III	Panel and Open Discussion Moderator: *A. Heyns* *No summaries available for this session*
Session IV	Transmissible Spongiform Encephalopathies Moderator: *J. Löwer*
Session V	New Safety Technologies II Moderator: *G.M. Fitzpatrick*
Session VI	Panel and Open Discussion Moderator: *R.Y. Dodd*
Session VII	Issues in Donor Recruitment and Selection Moderator: *A.E. Williams*
Session VIII	Paid vs. Voluntary Plasma Donation Moderator: *P.F. Strengers*
Session IX	Panel and Open Discussion Moderator: *L.A. Chambers*
Session X	Donor Management in the Development World: Challenges and Solutions Moderator: *J.-P. Allain*
Session XI	Movement Toward International Harmonization Moderator: *C. Smit Sibinga*
Session XII	Panel and Open Discussion Moderator: *J.S. Epstein*
Session XIII	Surveillance and Management of Medical Errors: Putting Data to Use Moderator: *R.M. Lewis*
Session XIV	Evidence-Based Transfusion Practice Moderator: *H.G. Klein*
Session XV	Panel and Open Discussion Moderator: *M. Brecher*

Preface

The International Association of Biologics (IABs) sponsored the first symposium on Advances in Transfusion Safety (ATS) in 1999 in collaboration with the University of California, San Francisco. Since then the biennial ATS Symposia have been held in 2001 at the Paul Ehrlich Institute, Langen, Germany, and in 2003 at the National Institutes of Health, Bethesda, Maryland, U.S.A. Under the leadership of Jay Epstein and Roger Dodd as the Co-Chairmen, working with the Scientific Programme Committee, the ATS-2003 Symposium was successful in bringing together worldwide experts in the field. This edited volume reflects the quality of their deliberations, now available to a wider scientific and medical audience.

For several years Professor Fred Brown, OBE, FRS (1925-2004) singularly edited the IABs Series – Developments in Biologicals with distinction and total dedication. His sudden death on 20th February 2004 caused an irreparable loss and a break in the tradition of timely publication of the proceedings of the IABs Symposia. Without much preparation we had to assume the responsibility for putting together the proceedings of ATS-2003. But for the help of Dr. Patricia Thomas and Catherine Vigny of IABs we could not have undertaken this daunting task. We hope this volume serves a useful purpose of being a ready resource for physicians and scientists interested in transfusion safety.

G.N. Vyas
University of San Francisco
San Francisco, CA, USA

A.E. Williams
Food and Drug Administration
Rockville, MD, USA

Contents

Vyas GN, Williams AE (eds): Advances in Transfusion Safety.
Dev Biol (Basel). Basel, Karger, 2005, vol 120, p 1.

SESSION I

Current Status of Blood Safety

Moderator: *J.S. Epstein*

Vyas GN, Williams AE (eds): Advances in Transfusion Safety.
Dev Biol (Basel). Basel, Karger, 2005, vol 120, pp 3-10.

Current Estimates of Transfusion Safety Worldwide

R.Y. Dodd

American Red Cross, Jerome H. Holland Laboratory for the Biomedical Sciences, Rockville, MD, U.S.A.

Abstract: Blood safety is a global public health priority. However, the degree to which blood is, or is not free of infection risk varies greatly around the world. The major determinants of this variation in risk are the availability of resources to support blood safety measures such as testing and the qualitative and quantitative epidemiological patterns of blood-borne infections. These factors are outlined and examples are presented.

Introduction

Many infectious agents are readily transmissible by blood transfusion. In most cases, the infectious agent has a prolonged, asymptomatic carrier state (for example, hepatitis B and C viruses, HIV, and the parasitic agents of malaria and Chagas' disease). However, it has recently become abundantly clear that some infections with a short, acute viraemia, such as West Nile virus, may also be readily transmitted by transfusion [1]. In the developed world, blood transfusion is extremely safe, particularly with respect to the risk of infection. Many measures contribute to this level of safety and there is a philosophy of continuous improvement and addition of new measures, such as nucleic acid testing (NAT). Many of these measures, although effective, appear to be beyond the normal bounds of cost-effectiveness [2]. In contrast, the developing world is generally unable to maintain a comparable level of blood safety as a result of very high prevalence and incidence rates for blood-borne infections and because of resource limitations.

Blood Safety Measures

Blood collection agencies use a number of processes to establish and maintain blood safety. These measures include (i) selection of low risk populations from which to solicit blood donors; (ii) careful screening and questioning of presenting donors;

(iii) quarantine of untested or suspect donations; (iv) laboratory testing of donations; (v) maintenance of records of prior donations and (vi) use of quality systems. While each of these measures is at least potentially available throughout the world, there are great differences in the extent to which they can be applied and in their efficacy.

Donor populations

In the developed world, the vast majority of whole blood donors are voluntary and non-remunerated. In addition, they tend to be drawn from a subset of the population with a somewhat higher level of socio-economic achievement, as measured by educational level and income. Additional measures that have been taken have been the elimination of collection of blood from certain institutionalized populations. All these broad selection measures were based upon epidemiological observations of increased infection risk from such populations. Voluntary donation is considered to be a necessary global standard by both the World Health Organization and the International Federation of Red Cross and Red Crescent Societies. The global distribution of voluntary, paid and replacement donors according to the Human Development Index (HDI) is shown in Table 1. It is clear that purely voluntary donations represent a minority (albeit of 31 and 40 %) in both low and moderate HDI countries. It seems encouraging that paid donations are reported to be an even smaller minority in these countries, with replacement donations making up the balance. Replacement donors are individuals who provide blood on behalf of an individual who is transfused. Conceptually, such donations are voluntary and the process appears to be a meaningful way to ensure that a safe blood supply is available. However, it transpires that not all such donations are, in fact, voluntary. In many instances, the replacement requirement is enforced so that patients are under considerable pressure to provide donors. At best, this results in a coercive situation, and at worst, it results in the use of so-called "professional" donors who are paid by the patient's family to provide the replacement donations. Thus, donations that are actually paid for may have been reported as "family/replacement". There are data that show higher frequencies of infectious disease markers among both paid and replacement donors in numerous different settings.

Table 1: Types of blood donations: Global distribution by Human Development Index (HDI).

	Low HDI number, (%)	**Med HDI number, (%)**	**High HDI number, (%)**
Volunteer	0.4m 31%	11.6m 40%	43.9m 98%
Replacement	0.8m 61%	11.7m 41%	1.0m 2%
Paid	0.1m 8%	5.6m 19%	0.03m NA
Total	1.3m	28.9m	44.93m

Some countries have developed approaches to stratify their donors for risk. For example, in Zimbabwe, a programme was established in which blood for transfusion was not collected from individuals without a recent history of prior donation, unless they were in the youngest eligible age-group. A creative concept has been to establish very safe donor populations through "donor clubs" as has been done in

Southern Africa. School age individuals are invited to join the club, which provides them with certain privileges and/or insignia and, in return, the club members pledge to give a certain number of donations during their membership. They also pledge to maintain a safe life-style. These programmes have led to donor populations with remarkably low risk for HIV, when compared to the general donor population in those countries [3].

Donor selection and screening

Presenting donors are usually interviewed to elicit medical and risk histories that are associated (or thought to be associated) with an increased likelihood of infectivity. Such interviews have become extremely comprehensive and taxing, involving around fifty separate questions in the U.S., and some of those questions may lead to further enquiry. It is important to understand that the origins and principal value of donor questioning relate to situations in which there was no other available intervention to reduce or prevent transfusion-transmitted infection. There is no question that the processes of donor selection and screening do result in the accepted donor population having materially reduced prevalence and incidence rates for key infections, when compared to those seen in the general population (Table 2).

Table 2: Prevalence and incidence rates, per hundred thousand – United States.

	Donor prevalence	Population prevalence	Donor incidence	Population incidence
HBV	1760 *	4900 *	3.0	111.4
HCV	299	1800	1.9	13.4
HIV	10	136	1.6	15.0

* HBsAg plus anti-HBc.

A key question is the extent to which such screening is of value in areas of limited resources and high rates of infection. At one level, questioning is a relatively inexpensive intervention. However, blood is a scarce resource and questions with poor specificity will unnecessarily reduce the number of available donations. Another point to consider is that any risk-based question must be based upon local epidemiological parameters. For example, it makes no sense to ask presenting donors about male-to-male sex if the predominant route of HIV transmission is heterosexual. Similarly, it is not necessary to ask about intravenous drug abuse in areas where it does not take place. A number of interesting sociological investigations have been undertaken in Zimbabwe, for example, and the findings of these studies have been applied to donor selection. In many cases, the outcomes are counter-intuitive to those schooled in North American and European practices [4,5]. The key message for transfusion services is that it is critical to understand the local epidemiological patterns of infections and the societal factors that contribute to their transmission, so that appropriate donor selection procedures can be designed.

Testing donations

The minimal global expectation for testing, as defined by the WHO, is that all blood for transfusion should be tested for anti-HIV, anti-HCV and HBsAg. While this standard has not yet been achieved, a great deal of progress has been made over the past few years. Dhingra reported that in low and medium HDI countries some 43 % of blood is not fully tested [6]. Table 3 indicates the extent of testing coverage in countries in South America in 1997 [7]. Clearly, significant improvements have been made since that time and most countries now report that 100 % of blood is tested for HIV. Such information may be found by searching at least some of the websites for WHO Regional Offices, using the term "Blood Safety". A potential problem with anti-HCV testing has been the high cost of the reagents, relative to those for HIV and HBsAg. Consequently, poorly resourced countries tend to perform less HCV testing. Compounding this basic difficulty is the problem of an assured supply of reagents. This becomes a particularly difficult challenge in countries with high inflation rates and correspondingly low currency exchange rates, as most reagents (and, indeed other supplies) must be imported.

Table 3: Range of testing coverage, prevalence and risk, Latin America, 1997.

		HIV	HBV	HCV	*T. cruzi*
Coverage:	High	100%	100%	100%	100%
	Low	100%	97.2%	25%	6.9%
Prevalence:	High	3.6/10k	10.2	8.5	37.3
	Low	0.7	1.5	1.3	1.3
Risk:	High	0/10k	0.7	12.3	83.7
	Low	0	0	0	0

Record keeping

A key to blood safety in the developed world is the ability to compare current test results with past results on the same donor. Not only does this provide a basis for error detection, but it is also used to prevent the use of donations from individuals previously found to be test-positive, or to have an unacceptable health or risk history. Such a process may have real value in countries such as the United States, where about 80 % of blood is collected from repeat donors. Clearly, computerized record systems also help. Although many blood systems in the developing world maintain excellent records, their overall contribution to safety would be restricted to regular donors.

Quality systems

The importance of quality systems cannot be ignored in maintaining blood safety. The use of such systems ensures proper management, consistency of practice and a culture of continuous improvement. Within the past few years, the WHO has included the need for quality systems to its key strategies for the development of transfusion services. To this end, it has established a global programme of quality training for blood programmes.

Factors Influencing Blood Safety

No matter how responsibly blood safety is managed, there are external factors that have a profound impact on the outcome of such programmes. Most important are the incidence and prevalence of transfusion-transmissible infections; and the adequacy of the available resources in a country or region.

Epidemiological issues

The epidemiology of blood-borne infections varies both quantitatively and qualitatively. It is unfortunate that the highest frequencies of these infections tend to occur in the areas of lowest resource availability. Furthermore, low resource countries have markedly reduced access to blood for transfusion. Indeed, 83 % of the world's population has access to only 40 % of the world's 75 million blood donations annually. In developed nations, there are about 40 to 50 donations for every thousand people, whereas in the least economically developed nations, the frequency is only one twentieth of that rate.

Globally, it has been estimated that there are about 42 million individuals living with HIV infection, 180 million with HCV infection and 370 million with HBV infection. These figures translate to global prevalence rates of 0.6 % for HIV, 3 % for HCV and 6.3 % for HBV. However, these rates are not evenly distributed and there are areas with HIV prevalence rates exceeding 20 %, HCV exceeding 10 % and active HBV infection greater than 8 %. Table 4 illustrates the number of individuals living with chronic, transfusion-transmissible infections by continent in 1998. While figures for HBV and HIV have probably not changed greatly, those for HIV have increased markedly (Fig. 1). In circumstances in which prevalence rates are high, testing results in the loss of a significant proportion of donations. In addition, such high levels of infection offer some risk, even in the presence of testing. Inadequate test sensitivity and the occurrence of test failures both offer greater risk in direct proportion to the prevalence rates. In addition, in areas of high prevalence, there is usually a high incidence rate. This generates a different risk, based upon the collection of blood during the seronegative, but viraemic window period that occurs during the early phase of infection.

Table 4: Estimates of subjects with chronic HIV, HCV, HBV infections, 1998.

Region	Population (millions)	Chronic infections (millions)		
		HIV	HCV	HBV
Africa	749	22.7	22.5	59.3
Asia	3,585	7.3	107.5	286.8
Latin America	504	1.7	15.1	10.3
Europe	729	0.8	21.8	10.9
Oceania	30	0.0	0.9	2.4
North America	305	0.9	9.1	1.9
Total	5,902	33.4	176.9	371.6

UNAIDS, WHO.

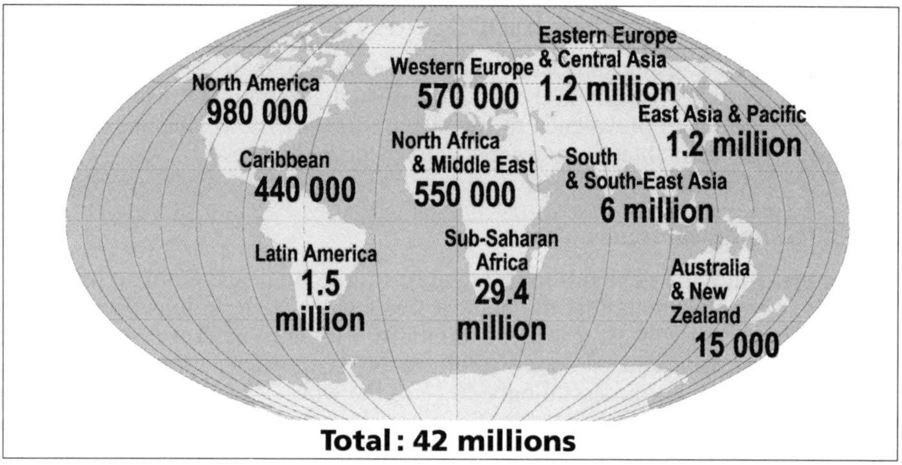

Fig. 1 : Adults and children estimated to be living with HIV/AIDS as of the end of 2002 (UN AIDS).

Epidemiological patterns of infection also have an impact on transfusion safety and need to be considered when considering donor selection methods. For example, while high school students are likely to represent a safer donor population, it is important to realize that in some sub-Saharan countries, the incidence of HIV infection increases earlier among girls than among boys. Thus, age and gender-specific selection criteria may need to be considered. In addition, as pointed out above, the pattern of transmission of infection needs to be well understood if effective donor questions are to be crafted.

Medical infrastructure

In many countries with a low HDI, the structure of transfusion medicine differs greatly from that in the developed world. There may be no organized blood centres and hospitals are responsible for collection and transfusion. In such environments, blood is often needed to treat anaemia of parasitism and blood loss during childbirth. The patient and the donor may present at the hospital at the same time, making it hard to perform all of the tasks necessary to ensure blood safety in a timely fashion. Alternate approaches to testing may be needed, including the use of rapid tests, or even pooled testing. Although these approaches are sub-optimal, it is important to recognize that any testing is better than none.

Examples

United States

Relative to many parts of the world, the United States has enviably low prevalence and incidence rates for transfusion-transmissible infections. The overall seroprevalence rate for HBV is 4.9 %, based upon measurement of HBsAg and/or anti-HBc, for HCV it is 1.8 % and for HIV, 0.14 %. Incidence rates are in the order of

0.1 % for HBV, 0.013 % for HCV, and 0.015 % for HIV. The corresponding prevalence and incidence rates for blood donors are much lower, indicating the impact of donor screening, which is based upon established risk factors. All whole blood donations are voluntary and non-remunerated and there are extensive testing programmes in place that include the use of nucleic acid testing for HIV and HCV. The residual risk of infection from the U.S. blood supply has been estimated at 1 in 205,000 to 1 in 488,000 donations for HBV, 1 in 1,935,000 for HCV, 1 in 2,135,000 for HIV and 1 in 524,000 to 1 in 2,993,000 for HTLV [8]. Similar data for other high resource countries have been published recently [9], in many cases, they illustrate a much lower risk than that estimated for the United States.

South Africa

South Africa is a resource-limited country with very high incidence and prevalence rates for HIV. It has a high-quality, independent blood supply system that is based upon free-standing blood centres. All donors are voluntary and non-remunerated. Risk factors are known and there are specific procedures to encourage self-exclusion by those at risk of HIV infection. There are creative approaches to donor management, including use of the donor club concept discussed above. The donor population has been evaluated for residual risk for HIV transmission on the basis of stratification into high- and low-risk populations. Among the high-risk populations, the prevalence of HIV infection is 4.9 % and the annual incidence rate is 0.5 %. In contrast, the low- risk population has a prevalence of 0.1 % and an incidence of 0.013 %. The corresponding residual transmission risk is 1 in 7,100 for high risk donors and 1 : 143,000 for the low risk donors. The overall residual risk is 1:28,400 [10]. Thus, even in an area with very high infection levels and a predominantly heterosexual transmission route, a high degree of transfusion safety can be achieved.

Argentina

Recent data are not available from Argentina. However, a recent publication did assess the risk of residual infection from blood donations in Argentina in 1997. Unlike the other studies cited, however, residual risk was assessed entirely on the basis of the proportion of blood that was fully tested. Thus, these data are illustrative only and should not be perceived as a statement of the current situation. Argentina is similar to many countries (particularly in South America), inasmuch as it has both private and public (i.e. government-operated) blood collection programmes. The former group had greater levels of testing coverage, at least in 1997. For the country as a whole, the risk of HIV infection was 1:16,400, for HBV, 1:8,100 and for HCV, 1:2,500 [11].

Measures to Improve Blood Safety Globally

There are many initiatives to improve blood safety. Some are necessarily limited and are directed to individual regions, countries or localities. It is not possible to comment on such programmes, other than to note that they all provide value and improvements. If they have a fault, it is that they tend to occur in isolation and may not be coordinated with broader efforts.

The WHO has an office devoted to blood safety. This office has initiated many important initiatives, including the development of basic expectations for the establishment and management of blood programmes, distance learning programmes, aides-memoires, information on the appropriate use of blood and, most recently, a comprehensive quality systems training programme. Additionally, many further blood safety programmes are initiated and managed through WHO's Regional Offices. Information about WHO's blood safety programme is accessible through their website : www.who.int.

One more initiative aimed at blood safety has been the establishment of the Global Collaboration on Blood Safety. (http://www.who.int/bct/Main_areas_of_work/BTS/GCBS/GCBS. htm) The Collaboration is a group of independent organizations that have interests and capabilities in blood safety. The GCBS mission and goals are (i) to promote and strengthen international collaboration on safety of blood and blood products and transfusion practices through (ii) improved collaboration among organizations, agencies and institutions involved in the safety of blood products and transfusion practices, with a view to (iii) encouraging and facilitating information exchange, (iv) promoting standards for good manufacturing practices for blood and related products for transfusion, (v) fostering the establishment of cooperative arrangements aimed at promoting the safety of blood donors and recipients in all countries, and (vi) promoting the safety, adequacy and quality of blood and blood products.

References

1 Pealer LN, Marfin AA, Petersen LR et al : Transmission of West Nile virus through blood transfusion in the United States in 2002. N Engl J Med 2003 ; 349 : 1236-1245.

2 Jackson BR, Busch MP, Stramer SL et al : The cost-effectiveness of NAT for HIV, HCV, and HBV in whole-blood donations. Transfusion 2003 ; 43 : 721-729.

3 Safe blood and safer sex. Education and counselling. AIDS Action 1996 ; 4-5.

4 Bassett MT, McFarland WC, Ray S et al : Risk factors for HIV infection at enrollment in an urban male factory cohort in Harare, Zimbabwe. J Acquir Immune Defic Syndr Hum Retrovirol 1996 ; 13 : 287-293.

5 Mbizvo MT, Ray S, Bassett M et al : Condom use and the risk of HIV infection : who is being protected ? Cent Afr J Med 1994 ; 40 : 294-299.

6 Dhingra N : Blood safety in the developing world and WHO initiatives. Vox Sang 2002 ; 83 Suppl 1 : 173-177.

7 Schmunis GA, Zicker F, Pinheiro F et al : Risk for transfusion-transmitted infectious diseases in Central and South America. Emerg Infect Dis 1998 ; 4:5-11.

8 Dodd RY, Notari EP, Stramer SL : Current prevalence and incidence of infectious disease markers and estimated window-period risk in the American Red Cross blood donor population. Transfusion 2002 ; 42 : 975-979.

9 Glynn SA, Kleinman SH, Wright DJ et al : International application of the incidence rate/window period model. Transfusion 2002 ; 42 : 966-972.

10 Fang CT, Field SP, Busch MP et al : Human immunodeficiency virus-1 and hepatitis C virus RNA among South African blood donors : estimation of residual transfusion risk and yield of nucleic acid testing. Vox Sang 2003 ; 85 : 9-19.

11 Schmuñis GA, Zicker F, Segura EL et al : Transfusion-transmitted infectious diseases in Argentina, 1995 through 1997. Transfusion 2000 ; 40 : 1048-1053.

Dr. R.Y. Dodd, American Red Cross, Jerome H. Holland Laboratory for the Biomedical Sciences, 15601, Crabbs Branch Way, Rockville, MD 20855, U.S.A.
E-mail : dodd@usa.redcross.org

Vyas GN, Williams AE (eds): Advances in Transfusion Safety.
Dev Biol (Basel). Basel, Karger, 2005, vol 120, pp 11-15.

Emerging Infectious Agents

D.A. Leiby

Transmissible Diseases Department, Jerome H. Holland Laboratory for the Biomedical Sciences, American Red Cross, Rockville, MD, USA

Key words: Emerging agents, blood safety, transfusion, transmission

Abstract: As new agents of infectious disease continue to emerge and old antagonists re-emerge, it is clear that the war on infectious disease is far from over. Indeed, the appearance of SARS during the past year is the latest example of the continuing challenges posed by agents of infectious disease. Emerging agents are threats not only to the general population, but also to recipients of blood transfusions. Today a variety of emerging agents are of concern to transfusion safety including *Trypanosoma cruzi*, West Nile virus, and *Babesia microti* to name but a few. These and other emerging agents have arisen or have been introduced partly through changes in donor demographics, international travel, microbial adaptations, land use, and human behaviour. Unfortunately, for many of these agents there is an absence of viable tests or other sound interventions to prevent their transmission at this time.

INTRODUCTION

During the 1960s, a de facto victory in the war on infectious disease was declared. The rapid implementation of new vaccines and antibiotic therapies promised to end the human suffering associated with infectious disease. However, the continued emergence of new agents and the re-emergence of old antagonists clearly demonstrates that infectious disease will plague humans for the foreseeable future. Indeed, the appearance of the SARS virus earlier this year represents the latest example of the many agents that have emerged during the past 30 years [1].

Emerging infectious diseases have been defined as clinically distinct conditions whose incidence in humans has increased during the past two decades [2]. Emergence can occur following the introduction or appearance of a new agent, the recognition of an existing, but previously undetected agent, or the reintroduction or re-emergence of an old agent. Multiple factors influence the emergence of infectious agents in human populations. Among these factors are changes in human demographics and behaviour, technology and industry, economic development and land use, international travel and commerce, microbial adaptation and change, and the breakdown of public health measures.

Emerging infectious agents also pose threats to blood safety, as shown by the emergence of HIV in the early 1980s. A variety of other emerging agents also pose blood safety threats (e.g., *Trypanosoma cruzi*, WNV, etc.). This review will briefly discuss several of these agents in the context of the factors that contributed to their emergence.

Changing Human Demographics

The emergence of several agents transmitted by blood transfusion has been influenced by changing donor demographics. Shifts in the demographics of the donor population have led many blood organizations to redirect recruitment efforts towards those groups currently under-represented in the donor pool. In some cases, this has led to an increase in donors at risk for infectious agents endemic to other parts of the world. Foremost among these agents are the *Plasmodium,* which cause malaria, and *Trypanosoma cruzi*, the aetiologic agent of Chagas' disease that will be discussed first.

T. cruzi is a small protozoan parasite endemic to Latin America, where an estimated 16-18 million people are infected [3]. Human infections are primarily acquired after exposure to an infected triatomine insect vector, but are also acquired congenitally, through organ transplant, or by blood transfusion. Infected persons generally experience a mild, acute disease lasting one to two months, followed by a lifelong asymptomatic indeterminate phase characterized by detectable antibody and intermittent parasitaemia. Later in life, 20-30% of infected persons will develop clinical Chagas' disease manifested by potentially fatal cardiac and gastrointestinal involvement for which drug therapy has limited effectiveness.

In the United States, 50,000 to 100,000 Latin American immigrants are thought to harbour chronic, asymptomatic *T. cruzi* infections potentially transmissible by transfusion[4]. During the last 15 years there have been seven reported cases of transfusion-transmitted *T. cruzi* in Canada (n=2) and the United States (n=5) attributable to donors born in *T. cruzi* endemic countries. These seven cases probably represent only the fulminate cases of disease since they occurred in immunocompromised patients; many more cases probably occur, but go unrecognized in immunocompetent blood recipients.

Estimates suggest that one in 25,000 U.S. blood donors is infected with *T. cruzi*; however, local infection rates can be much higher. In Los Angeles and Miami, seropositivity rates for *T. cruzi* were reported to be one in 7,500 and one in 9,000 blood donors, respectively [5]. Among directed donors the seropositivity rate in Los Angeles was one in 2,400. This same study indicated that the incidence of *T. cruzi* in Los Angeles blood donors increased significantly from 1996 to 1998, reaching one in 5,400 donors during 1998. This rapid increase in incidence was attributed to enhanced minority recruitment efforts necessitated by changes in donor demographics.

Like Chagas' disease, changes in donor demographics brought about by immigration have influenced the emergence of malaria as a blood safety threat. *Plasmodium falciparum*, *P. vivax*, *P. malariae*, and *P. ovale* are the aetiological agents of human malaria. These agents are found primarily in tropical and sub-tropical regions where they annually cause 300-500 million cases of malaria and 1.5-2.7 million deaths [6]. Humans acquire infection through the bite of an infected female anophelene mosquito, leading to invasion of erythrocytes by merozoites. High parasitaemias can lead to severe complications, including coma and death. Available drug treatments for malaria include chloroquine, quinine, doxycycline, and mefloquine for drug-resistant falciparum malaria.

In non-endemic countries, transfusion-acquired malaria is considered a rare event. Approximately one to two U.S. cases of transfusion-acquired malaria are reported annually, while Canada has reported only three cases in the last 10 years [7,8]. Implicated donors are usually asymptomatic or semi-immune persons who have visited an endemic country or emigrated to North America years earlier. Preventing transfusion-transmitted *Plasmodium* currently depends on obtaining an accurate donor travel history; however, misinterpretation of travel questions has led to several transfusion cases. Moreover, donor deferral due to travel history unnecessarily defers thousands of donors with minimal risk exposure, perhaps suggesting a need for testing. There is also an increasing possibility of malaria re-emerging in those non-endemic countries where competent anophelene vectors exist. The parasite could be reintroduced via the phenomenon of "airport malaria", but the more likely scenario for its re-introduction would be by an infected immigrant. Indeed, localized *P. vivax* infections were recently identified in suburban Washington, DC (2002) and Florida (2003) that were attributed to local mosquito populations acquiring the parasite from infected immigrants [9].

Microbial Adaptation, International Travel and Public Health Breakdown

The introduction of emerging agents to new human populations can also occur through microbial adaptation or international travel involving humans and/or animals. In many instances, once these agents have infected new populations their transmission is facilitated by breakdowns in public health. Certainly these factors have contributed to the emergence of West Nile virus (WNV) in North America. WNV is a flavivirus that was originally reported in the West Nile region of Uganda in 1937. Since its discovery, WNV has remained endemic to portions of Africa, Asia, Australia and Europe, where periodic outbreaks have occurred. However, beginning in 1999, an outbreak of WNV occurred in New York City that in subsequent years spread along the East Coast, into the South and Midwest, eventually pushing towards the West Coast in 2003. The virus is naturally transmitted among birds via culicine mosquito vectors, with humans serving as accidental hosts. In 2002, there were 23 cases of transfusion-transmitted WNV reported, several that resulted in deaths [10]. As a direct result of these transfusion cases, nucleic acid testing (NAT) was implemented in July 2003 to reduce the likelihood of transmitting WNV by transfusion.

Perhaps there is no better example of a disease that emerged as a result of international travel than severe acute respiratory syndrome (SARS). In November 2002, an apparently new human infection emerged near Guangdong, China that was subsequently spread across several continents by infected persons travelling on aeroplanes [11]. The SARS virus is spread by close personal contact resulting in an overall mortality rate of 15%, with a rate of 50% among elderly patients. The risk of transmitting the SARS virus by blood transfusion remains unclear. To date, there have been no reported cases of transfusion-transmitted SARS; however, to reduce the risk of transmission, blood donors in many countries were deferred based on travel to a SARS-affected area, contact with a known case, or a history of the disease itself. These interim measures were introduced pending the development of more information about the epidemiology, pathogenesis and transmissibility of SARS.

Changes in Human Behaviour and Land Use

During the past few decades humans have increasingly built homes in rural environments, reforested suburban neighbourhoods and greatly expanded their outdoor recreational activities. Taken together, these factors have all contributed to increased contact between humans and ticks, thereby facilitating the emergence of several tick-borne diseases.

Babesia microti is an intra-erythrocytic protozoan parasite that causes human babesiosis in North America. *B. microti* is transmitted to humans by *Ixodes scapularis*, the same tick that transmits Lyme disease and human granulocytic ehrlichiosis. Babesiosis usually presents as an asymptomatic or mild, self-limiting disease characterized by fever, headache and myalgia. More severe cases, particularly those in infant, elderly, immunocompromised or asplenic hosts, can demonstrate haemolytic anaemia, thrombocytopenia, renal failure and fatality rates approaching 5%. Babesial infections are usually treated with a combination of quinine and clindamycin or atovaquone and azithromycin.

Over 50 cases of transfusion-transmitted *B. microti* have been reported, including two cases involving the *Babesia*-like parasite WA-1, first described 10 years ago [12]. All transmission cases have been reported from the United States, with the exception of single transfusion cases reported in Japan and Canada. In virtually every transfusion case the implicated component was a red cell unit donated by an asymptomatic donor. The parasite can survive and remain viable in red cells for at least 35 days at 4°C, thereby enhancing the likelihood of transfusion transmission.

At this time, few interventions are available to control the transmission of *B. microti* by transfusion. Risk-factor questions concerning tick exposure have been shown to lack sensitivity [13]. The recent report of a specific and sensitive enzyme immuno-assay for *B. microti* suggests that a reliable and efficient blood screening test is feasible, but at present remains unavailable. With regard to window period infections, sensitive PCR assays for *Babesia* DNA suggest that nucleic NAT is also a viable option, particularly when coupled with serological testing.

Another emerging tick-borne agent of concern for blood safety is *Anaplasma phagocytophilum*, which causes human granulocytic ehrlichiosis (HGE). *A. phagocytophilum*, first described in 1994, shares a common tick vector (*I. scapularis*) and geographical range with the agents of Lyme disease and babesiosis. Symptoms of HGE are similar to those of other tick-borne infections; however, severe cases can be characterized by renal failure, gastro-intestinal bleeding, acute respiratory distress and death in 5%. Despite only recently becoming a notifiable disease in the United States, 351 cases of HGE were reported from a limited number of states during 2000 [14]. Seroprevalence and transmission data for *A. phagocytophilum* are limited, particularly among blood donors. Studies in donors from Connecticut and New York reported seroprevalence rates of 3.5% and 11.3%, respectively [12]. These reports, coupled with the survival of *A. phagocytophilum* in refrigerated blood for at least 18 days, and a reported transfusion case in Minnesota, indicates that this agent poses a potential blood safety threat [15].

Conclusions

Beginning with the reports of HIV in the early 1980s, new threats to the safety of the blood supply have continued to emerge every few years, including previously encountered or entirely new agents of disease. For most of these agents, epidemiological data regarding their prevalence and transmissibility is limited, thereby adversely affecting decisions regarding the implementation of appropriate control strategies. Only through continued surveillance and targeted research can we gain a clearer understanding of the blood safety risks these agents present.

References

1 Woolhouse MEJ: Population biology of emerging and re-emerging pathogens. Trends Microbiol 2002;10(Suppl):S3-S7.

2 Institute of Medicine: Factors in Emergence, in Lederberg J, Shope RE, Oaks SC (eds): Emerging Infections: Microbial Threats to Health in the United States. Washington, DC, National Academy Press, 1992, pp 34-112.

3 Anonymous: Chagas disease, Chile. Certification of interruption of transmission. Wkly Epidemiol Rec 2000;75:10-12.

4 Kirchhoff LV, Gam AA, Gilliam FC: American trypanosomiasis (Chagas' disease) in Central American immigrants. Am J Med 1987;82:915-920.

5 Leiby DA, Herron RM, Read EJ, et al: *Trypanosoma cruzi* in Los Angeles and Miami blood donors: Impact of evolving donor demographics on seroprevalence and implications for transfusion transmission. Transfusion 2002;42:549-555.

6 World Health Organization: World malaria situation in 1994. Wkly Epidemiol Rec 1997;72:269-276.

7 Mungai M, Tegtmeier G, Chamberland M, et al: Transfusion-transmitted malaria in the United States from 1963 through 1999. N Engl J Med 2001;344:1973-1978.

8 Slinger R, Giulivi A, Bodie-Collins M, et al: Transfusion-transmitted malaria in Canada. CMAJ 2001;164:377-379.

9 Malecki JM, Kumar S, Johnson BF, et al: Local transmission of *Plasmodium vivax* malaria – Palm Beach County, Florida, 2003. MMWR Morb Mortal Wkly Rep 2003;52:908-911.

10 Pealer LN, Marfin AA, Pertersen LR, et al: Transmission of West Nile virus through blood transfusion in the United States in 2002. N Engl J Med 2003;349:1236-1245.

11 Abdullah AS, Tomlinson B, Cockram CS, Thomas GN: Lessons from the severe acute respiratory syndrome outbreak in Hong Kong. Emerg Infect Dis 2003;9:1042-1045.

12 Leiby DA: *Babesia* and other parasites, in Brecher ME (ed): Bacterial and Parasitic Contamination of Blood Components. Bethesda, Maryland, AABB Press, pp 179-200.

13 Leiby DA, Chung APS, Cable RG, et al: Relationship between tick bites and the seroprevalence of *Babesia microti* and *Anaplasma phagocytophila* (previously *Ehrlichia* sp.) in blood donors. Transfusion 2002;42:1585-1591.

14 Summary of Notifiable Diseases in the United States, 2000: MMWR Morb Moral Wkly Rep 2002;49:x-xi.

15 Eastlund T, Persing D, Mathiesen D et al: Human granulocytic ehrlichiosis after red cell transfusion (abstract). Transfusion 1999;39(Suppl):117S.

Dr. D.A. Leiby, Transmissible Diseases Department, Jerome H. Holland Laboratory for the Biomedical Sciences, American Red Cross, Rockville, MD 20855, USA.
E-mail: leibyd@usa.redcross.org

Vyas GN, Williams AE (eds): Advances in Transfusion Safety.
Dev Biol (Basel). Basel, Karger, 2005, vol 120, p 17.

SESSION II

New Safety Technologies I

Moderator: *H.J. Alter*

Vyas GN, Williams AE (eds) : Advances in Transfusion Safety.
Dev Biol (Basel). Basel, Karger, 2005, vol 120, pp 19-24.

Bar Code Technology Improves Positive Patient Identification and Transfusion Safety

S.G. Sandler, A. Langeberg, L. Dohnalek

Departments of Pathology, Laboratory Medicine, and Nursing Services, Georgetown University Hospital, Washington, DC, USA

Key words: Blood transfusion, blood safety, bar code

Abstract: As a result of human error, an estimated 1 in 12,000 blood transfusions is given to the wrong patient. The cause of nearly all of these errors is failure of hospital personnel to identify positively intended transfusion recipients, their blood samples for cross-matching, or their correct blood components. We describe our experience using a point-of-care bar code transfusion safety system that links patients' bar-coded wristbands, with bar-coded labels on blood sample tubes, blood component bags, and nurses' identification badges. The result was 100 % accuracy of matching patients, their blood samples, and components for transfusions. For verifying information before starting blood transfusions, nurses preferred bar code "double checks" to conventional visual "double checks" by a second nurse. Methods are needed to reinforce nurses' proficiency with technological approaches to transfusion safety, such as software-driven bar code scanning, in situations where transfusions are administered infrequently.

Human errors that result in the "wrong blood" being transfused to the "wrong patient" may cause fatal haemolytic transfusion reactions, particularly when group A red blood cells are erroneously transfused to a group O recipient [1]. A study of 1,784,000 blood transfusions in New York State revealed 92 reports of erroneous transfusion (1 per 19,000) [2]. When these data are adjusted for under-reporting for ABO-compatible errors, the estimate of true risk of transfusion errors is 1 per 12,000 [2]. The most common errors are failure to ensure positive identification of patients, blood samples for compatibility testing, or blood components for transfusion. We first addressed this issue at Georgetown University Hospital in 1972 with the development of a prototype electronic patient-blood component identification transfusion system using a visual- and machine-readable hospital wristband along with a mobile device to transfer patient identification electronically to blood sample tubes and blood components [3]. While the system successfully provided the positive identification of patients, blood samples, and blood components, it was too cumbersome for routine hospital use and was not marketed commercially.

In 1998, we returned to the issue of positive patient identification in blood transfusion and conducted a study of a bar-code identification system in an outpatient transfusion service. That study used I-TRAC-Plus (Immucor, Norcross, GA) and demonstrated that a bar-code identification system could achieve 100 % positive identification for patients, blood samples, and blood components for transfusion [1,4]. Nurses preferred to perform conventional "double checks" for identification of patients and blood components using the hand-held data terminal/bar-code scanner compared to conventional visual "double checks" by a second nurse. We have transfused more than 1,000 blood components with this system, which currently functions as the routine "double check" for blood transfusions in this relatively high-volume outpatient nursing service.

The following report describes preliminary results of a new and continuing study of bar-code point-of-care technology for positive identification of patients, blood samples, and blood components for transfusion in an inpatient setting. The purpose of this second study is to determine whether nurses who transfuse blood relatively infrequently maintain proficiency and confidence using a bar-code system as readily as nurses who use the system frequently for transfusions.

Materials and Methods

MedPoint-transfusion bar-code system

For this second study, we selected MedPoint-Transfusion (Bridge Medical, Solana Beach, CA), a bar-code safety system that links patients' bar-coded wristbands with bar-code-labelled blood sample tubes and bar-code-labelled blood components for transfusion. An important factor in our selection of this system is that MedPoint-Transfusion is readily integrated with MedPoint-Medication, a companion bar code system for dispensing and tracking medications. We use a Symbol PPT 2800 (Symbol Technologies, Inc., Holtsville, NY) as the hand-held PC/bar-code scanner, although MedPoint-Transfusion's software operates on other pocket PC-based hand-held devices with radio frequency capability. The software program drives a series of bar-code identification checks for: (i) the operator's electronic signature (bar code on personal identification badge); (ii) the patient's name and medical record number (bar code on wristband); (iii) the blood component (bar code on compatibility label), and (iv) the blood centre's whole blood number (bar-code label on the blood bag). This sequence of prompts was designed to follow the customary "item-by-item" verifications required by the standards of the American Association of Blood Banks (AABB). [5]

Bar-coded wristband

The first step in our procedure is printing an eye-readable and bar-coded wristband using a dedicated PC and printer (Blaster Advantage, Cognitive Solutions) U.S.A.. Each wristband has three identifiers, e.g. the patient's first name, last name, and hospital medical record number (Fig. 1). Presumably, in a hospital-wide

Figure 1.

bar code transfusion safety programme, all patients would receive a bar-coded identification wrist band during the hospital admission process. Such procedures are already in effect in some hospitals, although not for transfusion-related purposes.

Bar-coded labels for blood samples

The next step is printing a bar-coded adhesive label for patients' blood sample tubes. To initiate this process, the software program directs nurses to scan their bar-coded identification badges and log-in by using personal passwords and the hand-held PC/scanner's keypad (Fig. 2). This procedure establishes an electronic signature for each transaction. Nurses then scan patients' bar-coded wristbands (Fig. 3). At this point, the program provides three options: (i) generating a blood sample label; (ii) initiating a blood transfusion, or (iii) recording

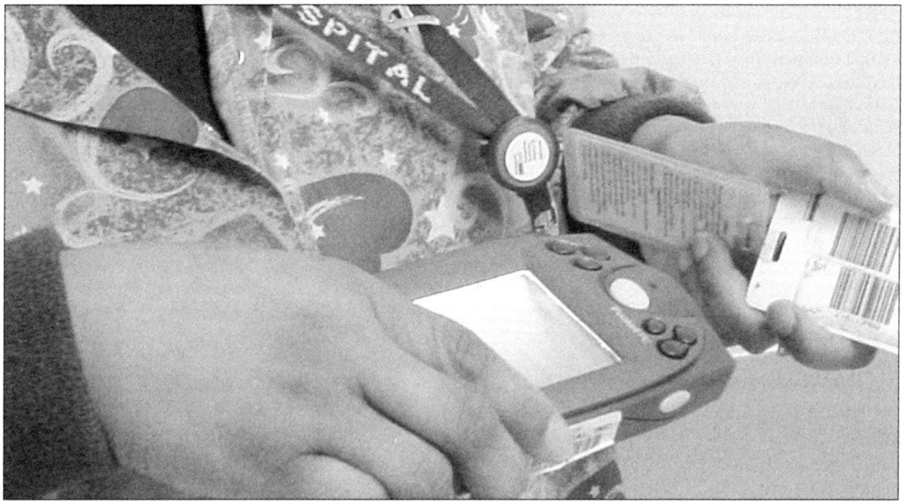

Figure 2.

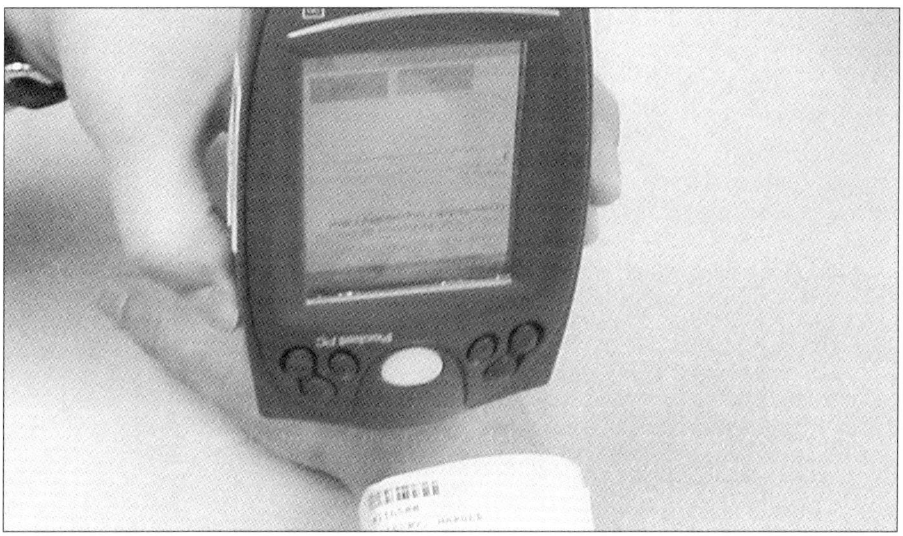

Figure 3.

patients' vital signs (not used for this study). After selecting the option to generate a bar-coded label for a sample tube, nurses are directed to align the PC/scanner with the radio frequency port of a portable printer (Zebra Encore 2, Zebra Technologies Corp., Warwick, RI) to generate two adhesive labels, one for a blood sample tube and another for the hospital's certification form. The first label contains the printed name of the patient, the date and time, the name of the person collecting the sample, the name of the test to be performed, and a bar code representing the patient's unique identifiers. The second label has the same information, without a bar code, to be attached to the certification form that will accompany the sample to the blood bank. Following collection of the blood sample – and while still at the patient's bedside – the nurse attaches the bar-coded label to the patient's blood sample tube and the second label to the blood certification form for delivery to the blood bank.

Blood bank testing

Upon arrival in the blood bank, patient's blood sample tube is inspected by a laboratory technologist for correct labelling and logged-in to the blood bank information system (Lifeline-Mediware Inc., Lake Oswego, OR), recording the requested services and the time of sample receipt. At Georgetown University Hospital, routine compatibility testing is performed using the ABS2000 automated blood typing analyser (Immucor, Norcross, GA) [6]. Samples are loaded in carriers and their bar codes are read by the analyser. When ABS2000 testing is completed, results are transferred to the blood bank's information system, reviewed by a technologist, and appropriate blood component units are selected from inventory for cross-matching (red blood cells) or issuing without further testing (fresh frozen plasma, platelets, cryoprecipitated AHF). After cross-matching, a bar-coded cross-match label is generated from the electronic records that contain the patient's name, medical record number, component code, and whole blood number. The cross-match label is attached to the back of the blood component bag. When a nurse requests a blood component for transfusion, a blood bank technologist issues the designated blood component by entering the request number attached to the unit. The technologist scans the whole blood number and the component code from the front of the blood component bag. This information is compared, visually, with the printed information on the label on the reverse side of the unit. At this time, the technologist performs a final visual inspection of the blood component for colour, clots, or other physical characteristics related to product safety and quality.

Transfusing blood components

To initiate the patient-component identification process for blood transfusions, nurses scan their bar-coded identification badges and enter their personal password in the keypad of the PC/scanner. Next, they scan the patient's bar-coded wristband and follow a series of screen prompts. The first prompt directs nurses to scan the compatibility cross-match label on the reverse side of the blood component bag that includes the patient's name, unique hospital record number, the blood component's code, and the patient's ABO/Rh type (Fig. 4). The

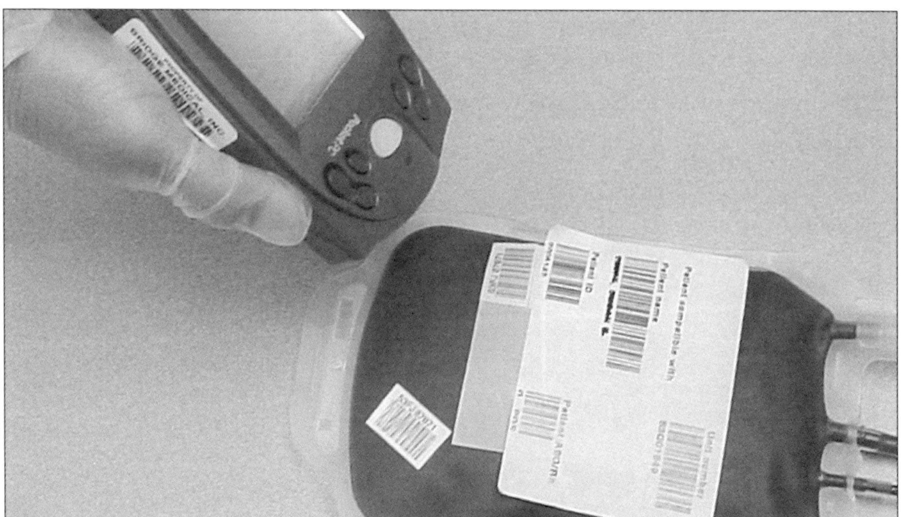

Figure 4.

next prompt directs scanning of the bar-coded blood centre's (donor) label on the front of the bag to verify that it matches the compatibility label. If all information meets the program's requirements, the PC/scanner signals to the nurse that the blood component has been properly matched for the patient and the transfusion is initiated. MedPoint-Transfusion's software has additional features that were not used in our study, including prompts for hospital-specific blood transfusion procedures such as confirming the expiry dates of the blood products, verifying physicians' orders for blood products, and validating that signed transfusion consent forms are placed in the patient's medical record. Also, the software can signal nurses to collect and record vital signs at hospital-designated intervals, but this feature was not used in this study. When not in use, the hand-held PC/scanner is returned to its cradle to recharge its battery and automatically download the record of transactions to the laboratory's dedicated MedPoint server. For this study, we use a Dell Server Pe350 (Dell Computer Corp, Round Rock, TX). However, the server can be any brand that meets MedPoint-Transfusion specifications. The capability of maintaining a centralized electronic record is an important feature of the MedPoint-Transfusion system, because it can capture and sort transfusion data by general categories (blood components, patients, nursing services) or other institution-specific categories for scientific, safety or operational analyses.

Training and in-servicing nursing staff

For this study, we selected an 18-bed high haematology-oncology-bone marrow transplant unit that is staffed by approximately 20 licensed registered nurses. Each nurse was trained during a one-hour session with an experienced user of the MedPoint-Transfusion system. The training session included a review of written materials and a step-by-step instruction on how to use the system. At the end of the session, all participants demonstrated proficiency with the MedPoint-Transfusion system. According to the hospital's Institutional Review Board-approved protocol, nurses were instructed to perform all aspects of the blood transfusion process, including identification procedures according to the hospital's standard operating procedures. Bar code identification checks using the MedPoint-Transfusion system were considered to be investigational procedures and were always conducted in parallel with the hospital's standard operating procedure. Nurses were instructed to alternate between performing a standard two-nurse visual "double check" first, followed by a bar code "double check" versus performing the bar code "double check" first, followed by the two-nurse visual "double check".

Results and Conclusions

Since October 2002, more than125 transfusions have been completed using the MedPoint-Transfusion system. Recruitment of patients for the study was interrupted for several weeks while we reinforced some process steps and awaited changes in the software program to accommodate suggestions from the participating nurses. All (100 %) patients, blood samples, and blood components for transfusion were positively and accurately identified. All (100 %) bar-code-labelled blood sample tubes and certification forms were legible with complete information. None of these samples was rejected or returned to nursing units because of illegible signatures, missing information, or mismatching information between sample tube labels and accompanying certification forms. The accuracy and reproducibility of information on bar-code-generated labels for tubes and forms is a major benefit in the blood bank, where as many as 15 % of hand written labels or forms may be returned because of illegible or imprecise information that does not meet strict blood bank standards.

Nurses' proficiency was 100 % using the bar-code system and confidence was high immediately following training. However, for some nurses infrequent transfusions and sporadic use the PC/scanner caused them to feel less proficient and confident than after training. Nurses who used the system less than twice weekly were inclined to feel less proficient and less confident after a few weeks had elapsed since training. We are currently analysing demographic characteristics of the nursing staff to ascertain if there are additional factors that are important for maintaining proficiency and confidence following training.

Conclusions

Bar-code technology offers a practical and efficient approach to improving transfusion safety by eliminating errors in identifying patients, their blood samples, and blood components for transfusion. MedPoint-Transfusion is a user-friendly bar-code system that is well-designed for meeting blood bank and regulatory requirements. It offers flexible formats for a wide range of hospital-specific procedures. The outstanding issue that requires further analysis is how to maintain nurses' proficiency and confidence using a bar-code identification system – or any other technological approach to transfusion safety – for nurses who transfuse blood infrequently. One approach could be "refresher aids," such as illustrated wall charts, to reinforce information learned during training. We have not studied whether using a similar bar-code system to dispense medications would have a beneficial impact on nurses using a bar-code system for transfusion safety. However, we would anticipate that simultaneous use of a similar technology for dispensing medication would be mutually reinforcing and increase the proficiency and confidence of users of both systems.

Acknowledgement

This project was funded, in part, by a grant from the Greenspring Financial Insurance Limited (GFIL), administered by the Risk Management Department, MedStar Health, Columbia, MD.

References

1 Sandler SG, Langeberg A: Technology can reduce errors in blood transfusion, in Lewis RF (ed): The impact of information technology on patient safety. Chicago, IL, Healthcare Information Systems Society, 2002, pp 57-66.

2 Linden JV, Wagner K, Voytovich AE, Sheehan J: Transfusion errors in New York State: an analysis of 10 years' experience. Transfusion 2000; 40: 1207-1213.

3 Chambers RW, Rubin MI, Rath CE, Sandler SG, Ball JH: A positive donor-recipient identification system for a regional blood transfusion service. Transfusion 1973; 13:34-36.

4 Sandler SG, Langeberg A, Berg M, Novak S: Decreasing the risk of transfusion-related human error by bar code identification of patients, blood samples, and blood components. Vox Sanguinis 2000; 79 (Suppl 1): abstract number 0138.

5 Menitove JE (ed): Standards for Blood Banks and Transfusion Services. 21st ed Bethesda, MD: American Association of Blood Banks. 1999, pp 52-53.

6 Sandler SG, Langeberg A, Avery N, Mintz P, the ABS Study Group: A fully-automated blood typing system for hospital transfusion services. Transfusion 2000; 40: 201-207.

Dr. S.G. Sandler, Department of Laboratory Medicine, Georgetown University Hospital, 3800 Reservoir Road, NW, Washington, DC 20007, USA.
E-mail: sandlerg@gunet.georgetown.edu

Vyas GN, Williams AE (eds): Advances in Transfusion Safety.
Dev Biol (Basel). Basel, Karger, 2005, vol 120, p 25.

SESSION IV

Transmissible Spongiform Encephalopathies

Moderator: *J. Löwer*

Vyas GN, Williams AE (eds) : Advances in Transfusion Safety.
Dev Biol (Basel). Basel, Karger, 2005, vol 120, pp 27-33.

Pathogenesis and Transfusion Risk of Transmissible Spongiform Encephalopathies

P. Brown

NINDS/NIH, Bethesda MD, USA

Key words: Transmissible spongiform encephalopathy, Creutzfeldt-Jakob disease, variant Creutzfeldt-Jakob disease, prion disease, transfusion risk

Abstract: The genesis (and pathogenesis) of sporadic and familial forms of human transmissible spongiform encephalopathy (TSE) is unknown, but the disease process may originate spontaneously in the brain as a statistically random event involving misfolding and amyloid formation of the " prion " protein. The pathogenesis of environmentally acquired TSE depends on the route of infection and is likely to involve both neural and haematogenous paths of neuro-invasion. Blood infectivity is well documented in experimental rodent models of TSE and in natural scrapie infections, but has not yet been proved to occur in humans. The knowledge that many plasma pools have included donations from individuals who later died of sporadic Creutzfeldt-Jakob disease (sCJD), together with the failure to identify any affected recipients, implies that the risk is either negligible or absent. In sharp contrast, two out of 26 recipients of labile blood products from individuals who later died from the variant form of CJD (vCJD) have became infected, and the still-living at-risk recipients are under continuing surveillance.

Transmissible spongiform encephalopathy was until the mid-1960s the exclusive province of veterinary medicine. Scrapie had been experimentally transmitted to sheep in 1936, and for the next 30 years was studied in sheep and goats, and then in mice, with most attention directed to defining the pathogenesis of disease and the nature of its causative agent. The landmark study of pathogenesis, which to this day stands as a model of its kind, was conducted by Dr. William Hadlow in a series of experiments involving hundreds of animals that were either sacrificed at intervals after birth (naturally occurring scrapie in sheep and goats), or after experimental infection (mice and goats) [1,2].

The general outline of pathogenesis was similar in each species: initial (presymptomatic) infection of the lymphoreticular system (and intestine in oral infection), followed by invasion of the central nervous system, and spread of infectivity to numerous peripheral organs during the clinical phase of disease. The ultimate distribution of infectivity is summarized in Table 1, which organizes a great deal of organ-specific data into a comparison of the range of infectivity levels in the central nervous system, lymphoreticular system, intestinal tract, and other tissues. Kimberlin later conducted numerous experiments designed to illuminate peripheral route(s) of neuro-invasion [3,4], and more recent studies, making use of the indicator "prion protein" PrP^{TSE}, have further refined the timing and spread of infectivity [5-7].

The experimental transmission of the human diseases – kuru and Creutzfeldt-Jakob disease (CJD) – obliged the research community to try and duplicate the same kinds of studies that had been carried out for scrapie, but time-course infectivity studies in humans were obviously impossible, and rodent and primate models of these human diseases have never received the same kind of attention lavished on scrapie. Nevertheless, these more limited data accord very well with the general schema of scrapie pathogenesis, as do data derived from a systematic study of bovine spongiform encephalopathy (BSE) (Table 2) [8]. It is curious, however, that whereas infectivity and/or PrP^{TSE} in cattle with BSE has a more limited tissue distribution than in any other animal or human form of TSE, infectivity/PrP^{TSE} in vCJD has a wider distribution than in other forms of human CJD.

Table 1: Range of infectivity titres (expressed as $\log_{10}LD_{50}/0.03$ ml) in tissues of animals at clinical stage of disease in natural and experimentally-induced scrapie. ic = intracerebral; sc = subcutaneous.

Donor species	Assay species	CNS	Lymphatic tissues	Intestine	Other tissues
Natural scrapie					
Sheep	Mouse (ic)	3.0-5.0	1.5-3.5	1.5-3.5	0-2.5
Goat	Mouse (ic)	4.0-6.0	2.0-4.0	1.0-3.5	0-1.0
Experimental scrapie					
Goat (sc)	Mouse (ic)	3.0-6.0	1.0-2.0	1.0-2.0	0-1.0
Mouse (sc)	Mouse (ic)	7.5	4.5-5.5	4.5-5.5	0-3.5

Table 2: Presence or absence of infectivity (bioassay) or PrP^{TSE} (Western blot or immunohistochemistry) in blood and "blood interactive" tissues of humans and animals with TSE.

Tissues	Human TSEs				Cattle		Sheep & goats	
	vCJD		Other TSEs		BSE		Scrapie	
	Infectivity	PrP^{TSE}	Infectivity	PrP^{TSE}	Infectivity	PrP^{TSE}	Infectivity	PrP^{TSE}
Spleen	+	+	+	+	-	-	+	+
Lymph nodes	+	+	+	-	-	-	+	+
Tonsil	+	+	NT	-	+	NT	+	+
Thymus	NT	+	NT	-	-	NT	+	NT
Lung	NT	-	+	-	-	NT	-	NT
Liver	NT	-	+	-	-	NT	+	NT
Kidney	NT	-	+	-	-	-	-	-
Bone marrow	NT	NT	(-)	-	+	NT	+	NT
Blood vessels	NT	+	NT	+	-	NT	NT	+
Blood	-	-	-	-	-	NT	+	-

The itinerary of the infectious agent within the body depends upon how infection is initiated (Fig. 1). In experimentally-induced rodent infections, when the agent is introduced by parenteral inoculation, neuro-invasion is preceded by a phase of replication within the lymphoreticular system followed by transport via the splanchnic nerve to the spinal cord [4]. In the spleen, mature follicular dendritic cells play an important role in replication, and maturation depends upon the presence of B-cells [9]. When the agent is given by mouth, positive immunostaining is first evident in lymphatic elements within the intestinal wall (M-cells and Peyer's patches) [10], and infection can by-pass the spleen to proceed directly from the gut to the brainstem via the vagus nerve [11]. The olfactory, optic, trigeminal, and hypoglossal tracts have also been identified as potential portals of entry [12-15].

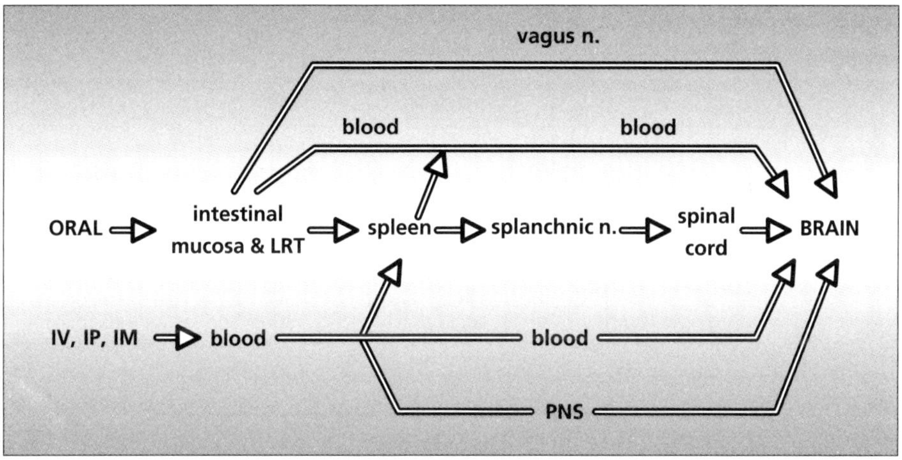

Fig. 1 : Neuro-invasive pathways from peripheral sites of TSE infection. The peripheral nervous system (with and without splenic involvement) has been well documented in experimental models. Haematogenous routes have been inferred to occur under some circumstances. IV = intravenous; IP = intraperitoneal; IM = intramuscular; LRT = lymphoreticular tissue; n = nerve; PNS = peripheral nervous system.

It is sometimes forgotten, in our enthusiasm for molecular biology, that the time-honoured infectious disease variables of dose and route of infection play a significant role in whether and when clinical disease will occur. High doses cause disease by both central and peripheral routes of infection, and tend to show similar incubation periods; low doses resemble high doses when given centrally, but show very long incubation periods after peripheral inoculation, and may not cause disease at all (Table 3). These characteristics were certainly critical in the outbreaks of iatrogenic CJD due to contaminated growth hormone and dura mater grafts, and are probably also important in the current outbreak of vCJD.

It may also be significant that clinical presentations following direct iatrogenic infections of the brain are indistinguishable from those of sporadic CJD, but different from those of iatrogenic disease caused by peripheral routes of infection. This difference suggests that the sporadic form of CJD may arise from within the brain itself, in which case infection would have no neuro-invasive phase. However, whether or not CJD arises from within, or there is blood stream neuro-invasion from without, is immaterial to considerations of risk: if blood is infectious at any point in the pathogenesis of the disease, it presents the same potential for iatrogenic transmission as any other circulating infectious agent.

Table 3: Influence of inoculum dose and route on incubation periods in non-human primates injected with either kuru or CJD titred brain tissue. ic = intracerebral; ip = intraperitoneal; im = intramuscular; sc = subcutaneous; iv = intravenous; id = intradermal.

Human case	Inoculated species	Inoculation route	Inoculum dose (LD_{50})	Incubation period (mths.)
Eir. (kuru)	Chimpanzee	ic	10,000	10
			10,000	11
			20,000	12
		ip, im, sc	75,000	18
		ic	30	15
		iv, ip, im, sc	50	142
Mat. (CJD)	Squirrel monkey	ic	20,000	16
		ic	20,000	18
		ic	10,000	20
		ic	20,000	30
		sc, id	80,000	24
		ic	200	18
		sc, id	800	no transmission

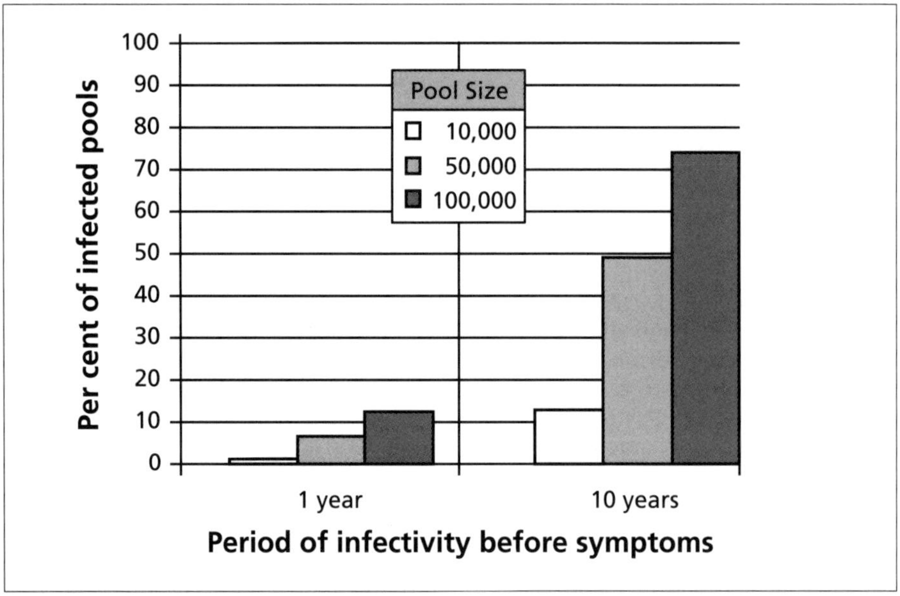

Fig. 2: Proportions of plasma pools containing contributions from at least one donor who later died of CJD, depending on the assumed period of pre-clinical blood infectivity (1 or 10 years) and plasma pool size (10,000, 50,000, or 100,000 units).

Although the few reported transmissions from the blood of patients with CJD have been questioned on grounds of non-reproducibility, and are far outnumbered by transmission failures, blood has been repeatedly shown to be infectious in experimental models of TSE, as well as in naturally occurring scrapie infections [16-19]. The chance that these data could also apply to human disease led regulatory agencies in the 1990s to promulgate industry guidance about destruction or at least quarantine of plasma products identified to have been "tainted" by CJD donor contributions.

Subsequent experiments showed that processing steps in the purification of most plasma derivatives reduce plasma input infectivity to levels well below what could ever occur in "tainted" plasma pools [20,21], and epidemiological investigations showed that despite the fact that a significant proportion of plasma pools included contributions from donors who later died of sporadic CJD, no case of CJD could be found among recipients of products derived from these pools. These three observations eased worries about the risk of transmissions via plasma derivatives therapy, but with the appearance of vCJD [22], the worries resurfaced because of: (i) uncertainty about the magnitude of the epidemic, and (ii) the presence of PrP^{TSE} in lymphoreticular tissues (not seen in sporadic CJD) – a combination that could augment the potential for contributions from donors incubating disease, and for blood to contain the infectious agent [23].

Epidemiological experience has borne out these concerns. Within the past year, two individuals with vCJD have been identified who had almost certainly become infected as a result of having received transfusions of packed red cells from donors who subsequently died of vCJD [24,25]. Records indicate that another 16 individuals are still alive more than five years after having received blood from the same donors (many others died of illnesses unrelated to CJD within a year or two of the donations), and another six to eight individuals are at similar risk from having received blood from two vCJD donors in France.

We cannot predict how many more at-risk recipients will succumb to this form of iatrogenic CJD, although experimental data suggest that the number may be small (Table 4). Similar transmission rates have been observed in sheep that were transfused with the blood of sheep with either experimental BSE or natural scrapie [19], and buffy coat specimens from four patients with vCJD failed to transmit disease by i.c. inoculation of RIII mice [26]. (This result was not unexpected because the "species barrier" effect would diminish the likelihood of disease transmission from samples with very low levels of infectivity).

The species barrier limitation was later avoided in an experiment using a murine model of vCJD [27]. Infectivity was detected in blood components of vCJD mice during both the pre-clinical and clinical phases of disease, but not at greater levels than in a non-variant model (GSS Fukuoka-1 strain). Other measures of virulence, including incubation periods, brain infectivity titres, and the accumulation of PrPres in spleens and brains, were also comparable in both experimental models.

Two other studies are still in progress. One is being conducted in cynomolgus monkeys, and the other in squirrel monkeys (Drs. C. Lasmézas and P. Brown, unpublished data). Methods include i.c. or i.v. administration of human vCJD blood components, and observation periods currently extend to between four and five years: no animal in either of the studies has yet shown signs of disease.

The similarities between blood transmission rates in experimental vCJD and non-vCJD animal models suggested comparable risks in humans and thus allayed fears that vCJD blood would pose any more danger than blood from donors who

Table 4: Blood infectivity levels or transmission rates in vCJD and non-vCJD models of transmissible spongiform encephalopathy. ID = infectious dose (the minimum amount of inoculum needed to transmit disease); ic = intracerebral; iv = intravenous

Donor	Recipient	Inoculum	Route of infection	vCJD/ BSE	non-vCJD/ scrapie
Mouse	Mouse	Buffy coat Plasma Whole blood	ic ic iv	20-30 ID/ml 20-30 ID/ml On test	30-50 ID/ml 10-20 ID/ml 1/20
Hamster	Hamster	Buffy coat Plasma Whole blood Whole blood	ic ic ic iv	- - - -	25 ID/ml 2 ID/ml 10 ID/ml 3/112
Sheep	Sheep	Buffy coat Whole blood	iv iv	1/7 4/11	4/11 3/10
Squirrel monkey	Squirrel monkey	Whole blood	iv	0/4	0/4
Chimpanzee	Squirrel monkey	Plasma Leukocytes	ic + iv ic + iv	- -	0/3 1/3
Human	Squirrel monkey	Plasma Buffy coat	ic + iv ic + iv	0/3 0/3	0/2 0/2
Human	Chimpanzee	Buffy coat Whole blood	ic iv	0/3 -	- 0/3

later developed sporadic disease, which was apparently nil. The occurrence of transfusion-associated cases of vCJD, in conjunction with these same experimental similarities, force us now to wonder if our failure to detect transfusion-associated cases of "sporadic" CJD may not be due to the difficulty of identifying such cases by virtue of the comparative frequency of sporadic disease coupled with the comparative infrequency of blood donations from older adults to adolescents.

References

1 Eklund CM, Kennedy RC, Hadlow WJ: Pathogenesis of scrapie virus infection in the mouse. J Infect Dis 1967; 117: 15-22.

2 Hadlow WJ, Kennedy RC, Race RE: Natural infection of Suffolk sheep with scrapie virus. J Infect Dis 1982; 146: 657-664.

3 Kimberlin RH, Walker CA: Pathogenesis of mouse scrapie: evidence for neural spread of infection to the CNS. J Gen Virol 1980; 51: 183-187.

4 Kimberlin RH, Walker CA: Pathogenesis of scrapie in mice after intragastric infection. Virus Res 1989; 12: 213-200.

5 van Keulen LJM, Schreuder BEC, Vromans MEW, Langeveld JPM, Smits MA: Pathogenesis of natural scrapie in sheep. Archives of Virology (Supplement) 2000; 16: 57-71.

6 Race RR, Oldstone M, Chesebro B: Entry versus blockade of brain infection following oral or intraperitoneal scrapie administration: role of prion protein expression in peripheral nerves and spleen. Journal of Virology 2000; 74: 828-833.

7 Brown P: The pathogenesis of transmissible spongiform encephalopathy: routes to the brain and the erection of therapeutic barricades. Cell Molec Life Sci 2003; 58: 259-265.

8 WHO Guidelines on Transmissible Spongiform Encephalopathies in relation to Biological and Pharmaceutical Products. Annex On line at WHO website: http://www.who.int/biologicals.

9 Brown KL, Stewart K, Ritchie DL, et al: Scrapie replication in lymphoid tissues depends on prion protein-expressing follicular dendritic cells. Nat Med 1999; 5: 1308-1312.

10 Beekes M, McBride PA: Early accumulation of pathological PrP in the enteric nervous system and gut-associated lymphoid tissue of hamsters orally infected with scrapie. Neurosci Lett 2000; 278: 181-184.

11 Beekes M, McBride PA, Baldauf E: Cerebral targeting indicates vagal spread of infection in hamsters fed with scrapie. J Gen Virol 1998; 79: 601-607.

12 Fraser H: Neuronal spread of scrapie agent and targeting of lesions within the retino-tectal pathway. Nature 1982; 295: 149-150.

13 Ingrosso L, Pisani F, Pocchiari: Transmission of the 263K scrapie strain by the dental route. J Gen Virol 1999; 80: 3043-3047.

14 Bartz JC, Kincaid AE, Bessen RA: Rapid prion neuroinvasion following tongue infection. J Virol 2003; 77: 583-591.

15 Zanusso G, Ferrari S, Cardone F, et al: Detection of pathological prion protein in the olfactory epithelium of sporadic Creutzfeldt-Jakob disease subjects. New Engl J Med 2003; 348: 711-719.

16 Brown P, Cervenáková L, McShane LM, Barber P, Rubenstein R, Drohan WN: Further studies of blood infectivity in an experimental model of transmissible spongiform encephalopathy, with an explanation of why blood components do not transmit Creutzfeldt-Jakob disease in humans. Transfusion 1999; 39: 1169-1178.

17 Bons N, Mestre-Frances N, Belli P, Cathala F, Gajdusek DC, Brown P: Natural and experimental oral infection of nonhuman primates by bovine spongiform encephalopathy agents. Proc Natl Acad Sci (USA) 1999; 96: 4046-4051.

18 Rohwer RG: Titer, distribution, and transmissibility of blood-borne TSE infectivity. Presented at Cambridge Healthtech Institute 6th Annual Meeting "Blood Product Safety: TSE, Perception versus Reality", MacLean, Virginia, February 13-15, 2000.

19 Hunter N, Foster J, Chong A, et al: Transmission of prion diseases by blood transfusion. J Gen Virol 2002; 83: 2897-2905.

20 Foster PR, Welch AG, McLean C, et al: Studies on the removal of abnormal prion protein by processes used in the manufacture of human plasma products. Vox Sang 2000; 78: 86-95.

21 Stenland CJ, Lee DC, Brown P, Petteway SR Jr, Rubenstein R: Partitioning of human and sheep forms of the pathogenic prion protein during the purification of therapeutic proteins from human plasma. Transfusion 2002; 42: 1497-1500.

22 Will RG, Ironside JW, Zeidler M, et al: A new variant of Creutzfeldt-Jakob disease. Lancet 1996; 347: 21-925.

23 Brown P: Variant CJD transmission through blood: risks to predictors and "predictees". Transfusion 2003; 43: 425-427.

24 Llewelyn CA, Hewitt PE, Knight RSG, et al: Possible transmission of variant Creutzfeldt-Jakob disease by blood transfusion. Lancet 2004; 363: 417-421.

25 Peden AH, Head MW, Ritchie DL, Bell JE, Ironside JW: Preclinical vCJD after blood transfusion in a PRNP codon 129 heterozygous patient. Lancet 2004; 364: 529-531.

26 Bruce ME, McConnell I, Will RG, Ironside JW: Detection of variant Creutzfeldt-Jakob disease infectivity in extraneural tissues. Lancet 2001; 358: 208-209.

27 Cervenakova L, Yakovleva O, McKenzie C, et al: Similar levels of infectivity in the blood of mice infected with human-derived vCJD and GSS strains of transmissible spongiform encephalopathy. Transfusion 2003; 43: 1687-1694.

Dr. P. Brown, 7815 Exeter Road, Bethesda, MD 20814, USA.
E-mail: paulbrown@comcast.net

Vyas GN, Williams AE (eds): Advances in Transfusion Safety.
Dev Biol (Basel). Basel, Karger, 2005, vol 120, pp 35-36.

Hemopure's Process Demonstrates TSE and Viral Clearance

A. Laccetti, J. Bagai, M.S. Gawryl, W.R. Light

Biopure Corporation, Cambridge, MA, USA

Background

Hemopure, for use as an alternative to red blood cells (RBC) in patients undergoing Orthopaedic Surgery, is a room temperature stable oxygen therapeutic developed to alleviate problems with RBC availability and oxygen transport to tissues. It does not require typing or cross-matching and transports oxygen to tissue more efficiently than RBC haemoglobin. Hemopure is a crosslinked formulation of ultrapure bovine haemoglobin and is produced in a GMP manufacturing facility by a 17-step purification and chemical modification process that has been studied for the removal or inactivation of potential pathogen contaminants.

Methods

Individual steps of the Hemopure process were evaluated for the clearance of six model viruses and two model scrapie agents (murine and hamster) for transmissible spongiform encephalopathy. Known titres of virus or scrapie agent were spiked into the initial starting material for unit operations (filtration, chromatography, or chemical addition) which were performed according to validated scaled-down procedures. An independent laboratory evaluated samples collected for viral and scrapie titre determination. Initial and final pathogen titres were compared to calculate clearance.

Results

The total log reduction (clearance) of six model viruses of different genome, family, size, and resistance to chemical inactivation, including two non-enveloped viruses, exceeded 16 logs for most of the enveloped viruses (xenotropic murine leukaemia virus, bovine viral diarrhoea virus, pseudorabies virus, and infectious bovine rhinotracheitis virus,) and 13 logs for the non-enveloped viruses (bovine parvovirus, and reovirus type 3). These clearance results surpass European Paul Ehrlich guidelines. The total reduction of a mouse-adapted scrapie strain as measured by *in vivo* assay in mice and a hamster-adapted scrapie strain as measured by Western blot assay was greater than 5.6 and 6.9 logs, respectively. Clearance was demonstrated by four steps for viruses including size and affinity separation and chemical inactivation, and two steps for scrapie including size and affinity separation.

Conclusions

The production process for Hemopure includes four steps relevant for virus inactivation or elimination and two steps relevant for elimination of TSE. The results indicate that Hemopure represents an extremely low and insignificant residual risk for viral or TSE infectivity in patients to whom it would be administered.

Dr. M.S. Gawryl, Biopure Corporation, 11 Hurley Street, Cambridge, MA 02141, USA.
E-mail: jclark@biopure.com

Vyas GN, Williams AE (eds): Advances in Transfusion Safety.
Dev Biol (Basel). Basel, Karger, 2005, vol 120, p 37.

SESSION V

New Safety Technologies II

Moderator: *G.M. Fitzpatrick*

Vyas GN, Williams AE (eds): Advances in Transfusion Safety.
Dev Biol (Basel). Basel, Karger, 2005, vol 120, pp 39-44.

Universal Pre-Storage Leukoreduction – A Defensible Use of Hospital Resources: The Yale-New Haven Hospital Experience

J.M. Fisk[1], *E.L. Snyder*[2]

[1] Division of Transfusion Medicine, Department of Laboratory Medicine, Yale New Haven Hospital, New Haven, CT, USA

[2] Yale University School of Medicine, New Haven, CT, USA

Abstract: In conclusion, as of 2004, it appears that in the United States in some hospitals, the use of LR blood products will probably remain as SLR rather than PSULR, due primarily to economic pressures. While some blood centres are slowly converting to ULR, there remains a mix of negative and positive feelings among physicians that make adoption of a national PSULR Standard of Care difficult. What is clear is that leukoreduction filters will cost more than the 170 um screen ("clot") filter. The use of PSULR to decrease the incidence of FNHTR, to decrease the incidence of HLA alloimmunization, and its use in lieu of CMV-seronegative blood products is well supported in the medical literature. However, this issue will probably continue to be revisited and debated for some time before a national standard policy for PSULR is adopted. Finally, we believe that despite increasing economic pressures and worsening budgetary constraints, the decision to adopt PSULR should rest primarily on medical reasons: as a means of improving patient care. In the view of the authors, pre-storage universal leukoreduction qualifies as a significant and medically justifiable improvement in the care of all hospital patients.

Leukoreduction

Leukoreduction refers to the process of lowering the concentration of passenger leukocytes in blood components with the intention of reducing the incidence of complications from recipient exposure to high levels of donor white blood cells. In practice, this is usually accomplished using 3rd generation leukoreduction filters that are capable of attaining a 4-log_{10} reduction in leukocyte concentration. Thus, $\leq 5 \times 10^6$ leukocytes are infused during transfusion of a unit of Red Blood Cells, Single Donor Platelets, or a pool of Whole Blood Platelet Concentrates. Leukoreduction may be performed at the blood collection centre as part of pre-storage processing under U.S. Food and Drug Administration (FDA) current Good Manufacturing Practices (cGMP) guidelines, at the bedside during blood component transfusion using in-line leukoreduction filters, or by in-process leukoreduction during plateletpheresis by automated apheresis collection instruments. Leukoreduction as part of transfusion practice may be either selective (SLR) or universal (ULR). SLR generally occurs at the request of the physician caring for a patient or at the discretion of the medical director of the blood bank. The degree to which SLR is used depends primarily on the identification of a selected group of patients deemed most likely to benefit from reduced donor leukocyte exposure. This includes patients such as potential bone marrow transplant recipients or patients with a history of recurrent febrile non-haemolytic transfusion reactions. ULR, in contrast, provides benefit to all patients including those without a specific indication. The decision to adopt a ULR must weigh the benefit of improved patient care against the cost of resource use coupled with budgetary constraints.

Leukoreduction Policies at Yale-New Haven Hospital

In April, 1999 following the approval of the Yale-New Haven Hospital (YNHH) Transfusion Committee, the Hospital Medical Board ratified a proposal from the Blood Bank Director (ELS) to switch to 100 % Prestorage Universal Leukoreduction (PSULR) of all Red Blood Cells, Whole Blood Platelet Concentrates, and Platelets Apheresis units. This proposal was agreed upon by the hospital's sole-source blood supplier: the Connecticut region of the American Red Cross. Yale-New Haven Hospital is a university-affiliated, 900 + bed tertiary care facility with a yearly (2002 data), blood product transfusion level of approximately 20,000 Red Blood Cells (RBC), 15,000 Random Donor Platelets (RDP), and 100 Single Donor Platelets (SDP). Before 1998, SLR was performed at the bedside in approximately 20-30 % of transfusion cases. After the decision was made to adopt a policy of 100 % PSULR, a six to eight month transition period was needed before full conversion was realized. Driving this decision was the conviction that PSULR provided tangible and significant improvements in patient care, particularly to certain high-risk populations cared for at the hospital, which included oncology, stem cell transplant, chronically anaemic, solid organ transplant, and high risk obstetrical patients. Offsetting this was an appreciation of the financial impact that this decision would have, coupled with an acknowledgement that the blood bank, despite its role as a provider of a vital medical service, remained an administrative cost centre.

Budgetary and Funding Considerations

At its inception, establishment of PSULR resulted in an increased annual expenditure of approximately $300,000, representing 3.8 % of the blood bank budget and 0.06 % of the total hospital budget. This increase, while substantial, was kept as low as possible by use of cost-saving strategies (identified by an *) seen in Table 1. Several strategies proved particularly beneficial. Immediate cost savings were realized from the elimination of both routine CMV serological testing that had been provided for all patients with malignancies and the use of bedside leukoreduction filters throughout the hospital (cost shifting). Conversion to 100 % PSULR also obviated the need for maintaining dual inventories of CMV-seronegative and CMV-untested blood products. This resulted in a significant and durable decrease

Table 1: Strategies for introducing new technologies*

1. Link new technology advances with Federal or State regulatory requirements
2. * Incremental incorporation strategy, i.e. step-up introduction of new technology
3. * Internally reallocate funds (a.k.a. "cost shifting")
4. Link new technology advances to their implementation or adoption at peer institutions
5. * Consider cost savings from dose management (such as smaller platelet pool size or more stringent transfusion guidelines)
6. * Link new technology advances to decreased FTEs (personnel)
7. Link new technology advances to strong clinical service and improved patient care and outcomes
8. Obtain support from Risk Management

* signifies cost-saving strategies

in the outdating and wastage of platelets: from 13 % during SLR to 4.8 % after adoption of PSULR. This led to even greater cost savings as fewer platelet units were outdated and wasted. Although the effect on outdating and wastage of red blood cell units was minimal (<0.5%), it nonetheless provided some additional cost savings.

Concurrent with the implementation of PSULR were shifts in transfusion guidelines to bring practices into line with the latest research findings on best transfusion practice. This resulted in an overall decrease in red blood cell and platelet use as in-patient transfusion thresholds were lowered (the platelet "trigger" was decreased from < 20,000/μL to < 10,000/μL), the platelet pool size was decreased from five-unit pools to four-unit random donor platelet pools for in-patients; single-unit (rather than two- unit) red blood cell transfusion was encouraged for elective transfusion of anaemic patients.

In concert, these interventions brought the incremental cost of 100 % PSULR of red blood cells and platelets down to approximately $300,000 annually, while improving transfusion practice, establishing an inventory composed solely of CMV-safe products, and decreasing blood product wastage. Overwhelming benefits were also seen in an improvement in patient care that was realized in three principal areas:

(i) a decreased incidence of Human Leukocyte Antigen (HLA) alloimmunization;

(ii) a decreased incidence of Febrile Non-haemolytic Transfusion Reactions (FNHTR);

(iii) a continuation of a lack of reported transfusion-transmitted cytomegalovirus (TT-CMV) infections.

Reduction in HLA Alloimmunization

The role of leukoreduction in reducing the incidence of HLA alloimmunization was well established by the Trial to Reduce Alloimmunization to Platelets [1] (TRAP Study). This prospective, multi-institutional, randomized, and blinded trial attempted to evaluate the relative efficacy of three approaches to alloimmunization prophylaxis: leukofiltration of pooled random donor platelet (RDP) concentrates, UV-B irradiation of pooled RDP concentrates, and use of filtered apheresis platelet (F-AP) units from random donors. All three treatment arms were statistically significantly better than the control arm for the study endpoints of alloimmune platelet refractoriness, platelet refractoriness, and LCA positivity; no appreciable difference existed among the three treatment arms for any of these endpoints. Interestingly, no additional benefit was gained from the use of leukoreduced single donor apheresis platelet units compared to leukoreduced pooled random donor whole blood platelet concentrates.

To date, there has been no refutation of this work despite certain limitations. These aspects include the fact that the leukoreduction filters available at the time of the study provided only a 3-$\log_{10}$ reduction in white blood cells compared with the current generation of filters capable of an additional log order reduction, and the fact that between 3-5 % of the reported transfusions were "off-protocol". Recently, a large retrospective study was published by Seftel et al [2] involving analysis of 13,902 platelet transfusions in 617 patients undergoing chemotherapy for acute leukemia or stem cell transplantation before (n = 315) and after (n = 302) the introduction of universal leukoreduction (ULR) by the Canadian Blood Services. They found that alloimmunization and alloimmune platelet refractoriness was significantly ($P < 0.001$) reduced in the post-ULR group, and that the post-ULR group required far fewer HLA-matched platelets ($P < 0.001$). These studies provide compelling evidence for the effectiveness of PSULR in preventing HLA alloimmunization, its attendant post-transfusion complications and a potentially costly requirement for HLA-matched platelets.

Reduction in the Incidence of Febrile Non-haemolytic Transfusion Reactions (FNHTR)

A second significant benefit to the use of PSULR blood products is a reduction in FNHTR, a phenomenon that has been the subject of much investigation at our institution. The results of this retrospective investigation were recently published by Paglino et al [3] in which a total of 145,369 red blood cell and 137,982 platelet concentrate transfusions were analysed during the period of January 1995 to December 2002. The rates of FNHTR and allergic transfusion reactions (ATR) were ascertained for the periods of selective leukoreduction (SLR) and the subsequent institution of universal leukoreduction (PSULR). For red blood cells, the relative FNHTR rate fell 47.1 % (from 0.34 % (SLR) to 0.18 % (PSULR); $P < 0.0001$) and for platelets, the relative FNHTR rate fell 93.1 % (from 2.18 % (SLR) to 0.15 % (PSULR); $P < 0.0001$). No statistically significant change in the rate of allergic reactions for red blood cell or platelet transfusion was detected. A chart review of 500 patients receiving transfusion – 300 patients receiving red blood cells and 200 patients receiving platelets – all without report of a reaction, was undertaken to determine whether there was an appreciable rate of under-reporting of reactions. Of these 500 patients, only one patient had a fever to 100.2° F that was not reported, supporting the conclusion that the decrease in the rate of FNHTR was not due to nursing inattention.

These findings are in general agreement with rates published in numerous recent studies [4-9], although other investigators [10,11] have found no change in the rate of post-ULR FNHTR. The weight of current evidence, thus, appears to support the conclusion that ULR results in a decrease in febrile reactions to both red blood cells and platelets. Further, no study to date has been able to link irrefutably the use of PSULR to other outcome measures such as decreased length-of-stay (LOS), decreased antibiotic usage, or lowered rates of infection.

Reduction in Transfusion-Transmitted Cytomegalovirus (TT-CMV) Infection

A final compelling benefit to the adoption of PSULR is its effect on the rate of transfusion-transmitted CMV (TT-CMV) infection, although this remains a controversial, and at times a hotly debated topic. What is well established is that there are well-defined patient groups for whom the risk of CMV infection and disease is known. These include:

(i) CMV-seronegative pregnant women;

(ii) premature infants (<1200 g) born to a CMV-seronegative mother;

(iii) CMV-seronegative recipients of allogeneic bone marrow transplants from CMV-seronegative donors;

(iv) CMV-seronegative patients with AIDS.

A longstanding dictum is that these patients should be supported solely by use of CMV-seronegative blood products due to the potentially devastating complications of primary CMV infection and disease in these populations. One of the first studies to challenge this view was published by Bowden et al [12]. They found that 3rd generation leukofiltered blood was as effective as CMV-seronegative blood for the prevention of TT-CMV infection in CMV-seronegative bone marrow transplant recipients following transplantation. They found that survival at day 100 for patients receiving filtered blood was equal to that of the group receiving screened, CMV-seronegative blood. This work was subsequently cited as providing a rational basis for recommendations published in the Guidelines for Preventing Opportunistic Infections In Hematopoietic Stem Cell Transplant Recipients [13], a consensus set of recommendations from the United States Center for Disease Control (CDC), the Infectious Disease Society of America, and the American Society of Blood and Marrow Transplantation.

Despite this, there remains some debate in the medical literature as to the equivalence of leukoreduced (CMV-safe) and CMV-seronegative blood products. A report by Nichols et al [14] found an increased rate of CMV infection after institution of leukocyte-reduced apheresis platelet usage at their institution. Interestingly, they found that the administration of filtered red blood cell products, but not apheresis platelets products, from CMV-seropositive donors was the primary predictor of TT-CMV. Numerous studies [15-17], however, continue to support the use of leukoreduced blood products as CMV-safe in high-risk patient populations. At present, the U.S. FDA Guidance for Industry supports the tenet that PSULR blood products "contribute to safety" (as per two BPAC meetings) and the benefits of increased safety should prompt blood suppliers to make them more widely available. It further stipulates that PSLR may be used in lieu of CMV serological testing as a means of rendering blood components "CMV-safe".

REFERENCES

1 The Trial To Reduce Alloimmunization To Platelets Study Group: Leukocyte Reduction and Ultraviolet B Irradiation of Platelets to Prevent Alloimmunization and Refractoriness to Platelet Transfusions. N Engl J Med 1997; 337: 1861-1869.

2 Seftel MD, Growe GH, Petraszko T, Benny WB, Le A, Lee C, Spinelli JJ, Sutherland HJ, Tsang P, Hogge DE: Universal prestorage leukoreduction in Canada decreases platelet alloimmunization and refractoriness. Blood 2004; 103: 333-339.

3 Paglino JC, Pomper GJ, Fisch GS, Champion MH, Snyder EL: Reduction of febrile but not allergic reactions to RBCs and platelets after conversion to universal prestorage leukoreduction. Transfusion 2004; 44: 16-24.

4 Serinolli MI, Novaretti MCZ, Dorlhiac-Llacer PECD: Comparison of allergic and febrile non-hemolytic transfusion reactions in recipients of buffy-coat or non-buffy-coat reduced red blood cell concentrates (abstract). Transfusion 2002; 42 (Suppl): 21S.

5 Andreu G, Morel P, Forestier F, et al: Hemovigilance network in France: organization and analysis of immediate trans-fusion incident reports from 1994 to 1998. Transfusion 2002; 42: 1356-1364.

6 Landmark J, Schafer D, Warkentin PI: Effect of universal pre-storage leukocyte-reduced transfusions on transfusion reaction rates in a tertiary care hospital (abstract). Transfusion 2001; 41 (Suppl): 113S.

7 Sweeney JD: Decrease in reaction rates after implementing universal leukoreduction (abstract). Transfusion 2001; 41 (Suppl): 112S.

8 King KE, Shirey RS, Thoman SK, et al: Universal leukoreduction decreases the incidence of febrile non-hemolytic transfusion reactions to RBCs Transfusion 2004; 44: 25-29.

9 Yazer MH, Podlosky L, Clarke G, Nahirniak SM: The effect of prestorage WBC erduction on the rates of febrile nonhemolytic transfusion reactions to platelet concentrates and RBC. Transfusion 2004; 44: 10-15.

10 Dzik WH, Anderson JK, O'Neill EM, et al: A prospective, randomized clinical trial of universal WBC reduction. Transfusion 2002; 42: 1114-1122.

11 Becker JL, Boyd JC, Mintz PD: Febrile non-hemolytic transfusion reactions reported in patients receiving prestorage leukocyte-reduced or non-leukocyte reduced red blood cells or apheresis platelets (abstract). Transfusion 2001; 41 (Suppl): 112S.

12 Bowden RA, Slichter SJ, Sayers M, et al: Comparison of filtered leukocyte-reduced and cytomegalovirus (CMV) seronegative blood products for the prevention of transfusion-associated CMV infection after marrow transplant. Blood 1995; 86: 3598-3603.

13 Centers for Disease Control: Infectious Diseases Society of America, American Society for Blood and Marrow Transplantation. Guidelines for preventing opportunistic infections among hematopoietic stem cell transplant recipients. Biol Blood Marrow Transplantation 2000; 6: 659-734.

14 Nichols WG, Price TH, Gooley T, et al: Transfusion-transmitted cytomegalovirus infection after receipt of leukoreduced blood products. Blood 2003; 101: 4195-4200.

15 Zaia JA: Prevention of cytomegalovirus disease in hematopoietic stem cell transplantation. Clin Infect Dis. 2002; 35: 999-1004.

16 Boeckh M, Nichols WG, Papanicolaou G, Rubin R, Wingard JR, Zaia J: Cytomegalovirus in hematopoietic stem cell transplant recipients: Current status, known challenges, and future strategies. Biol Blood Marrow Transplant 2003; 9: 543-558.

17 Blajchman MA, Goldman M, Freedman JJ, Sher GD: Proceedings of a consensus conference: prevention of post-transfusion CMV in the era of universal leukoreduction. Transfus Med Rev 2001; 15:1-20.

Dr. E.L. Snyder, Yale University School of Medicine, 333 Cedar Street, New Haven, CT 06510, USA.
E-mail: edward.snyder@yale.edu

Vyas GN, Williams AE (eds): Advances in Transfusion Safety.
Dev Biol (Basel). Basel, Karger, 2005, vol 120, pp 45-52.

Blood Substitutes: How Close to a Solution?

H.G. Klein

Department of Transfusion Medicine, Warren G. Magnuson Clinical Center, National Institutes of Health, Bethesda, MD, U.S.A.

Abstract: The term "blood substitute" is commonly misused when "red cell substitute (RCS) is meant. The ideal RCS should deliver (i) oxygen; (ii) require no compatibility testing; (iii) cause few side effects; (iv) have prolonged storage qualities; (v) persist in the circulation and (vi) be available at reasonable cost. While no drug with all these qualities is on the near horizon, several early generation RCS are approaching submission for licensing, at least for limited indications. Haemoglobin-derived RCS from human, bovine and recombinant sources, as well as perfluorochemicals that dissolve O2 are in different stages of development. While each formulation has its own physical characteristics, biological activities, and adverse reaction profile, all share one characteristic: the physiological consequences of delivering O2 with small molecules is poorly understood and may both account for problems seen in the clinical trials and provide therapeutic opportunities for the cancer patient. Those RCS in phase III trials all have a half-life measured in hours and are unlikely to replace transfusions or drugs that stimulate erythropoiesis for chronic anaemia, but they may play a role (i) in military and civilian trauma as resuscitation solutions, (ii) as a bridge to transfusion when no compatible blood is immediately available, (iii) as an adjunct to the autologous haemodilution management of surgery, or even (iv) in radiation therapy or the management of cancer-related vascular occlusive syndromes.

Introduction

Early transfusion history described the miraculous recovery of patients suffering life-threatening haemorrhage. However, equally dramatic reports revealed unexpected, unexplained, and occasionally lethal complications. The emergence of HIV as a transfusion-transmitted virus was only the latest of such complications and certainly will not be the last. Little wonder that the medical establishment, the public and, more recently, the biotechnology industry, place such high hopes on the development of safer alternatives to blood. Despite more than 40 years of focused research, and the recent infusion of hundreds of millions of venture capital dollars, no credible replacement for blood has yet been approved for use in the United States. That may soon change.

This article was written in a personal capacity and does not necessarily represent the opinions of the NIH, DHHS or the Federal Government.

The term "blood substitute" is a misnomer. So-called blood substitutes in fact replace only one or possibly two functions of transfused blood. By this definition, several blood substitutes are already in common use: dextran and starch solutions that act as volume expanders, recombinant proteins that replace, among other things, coagulation factors, and even anticoagulants such as warfarin and heparin that are used on occasion to substitute for naturally occurring anticoagulant proteins. For other functions of blood, those of platelets and leukocytes, no substitute is likely to emerge in the near future. However the "holy grail" of blood substitute research has been to develop a red cells substitute (RCS), a small molecule that (i) delivers oxygen efficiently; (ii) requires no compatibility testing; (iii) can be sterilized; (iv) has a long shelf-life at room temperature; (v) reconstitutes easily; (vi) persists in the circulation for days or weeks and (vii) can be provided at a price competitive with that of human blood. While no such substance is on the near horizon, several candidate agents with several of these qualities are undergoing clinical trials.

Candidate RCS fall into three general classes, perfluorochemicals (PFC), haemoglobin-based oxygen carriers (HBOC), and liposome-encapsulated haemoglobin. Although it is convenient to review these drugs as "classes," each formulation should be considered a unique drug with its own physical characteristics, biological activities, and adverse reaction profile. General characteristics of these classes are reviewed in Tables 1 and 2.

Perfluorochemical Emulsions

Perfluorochemicals are synthetic, inert, hydrophobic molecules with an almost unlimited ability to dissolve gases, including oxygen. Because these molecules are structurally similar to hydrocarbons, they are not water-soluble and therefore must be emulsified with surfactants before they are suitable for intravenous use. This

Table 1: Features of oxygen carrier classes.

Haemoglobin-based	Perfluorochemical
1. physiological O2 carrier characteristic	1. process controlled manufacture
2. lack red cell antigens	2. sterile
3. potential high oncotic pressure	3. minimal immunogenicity
4. long shelf-life	4. long shelf-life
5. protein pathogen inactivation possible	5. inexpensive

Table 2: Limitations of oxygen carriers.

Haemoglobin-based	Perfluorochemical
1. rapid clearance	1. rapid clearance
2. auto-oxidation	2. emulsification/storage
3. vaso-activity	3. long tissue persistence
4. potential immunogenicity	4. requires supplemental O2
5. expensive	5. side effects

property has complicated their preparation and storage and the nature of the emulsifier turns out to be as important as the perfluorochemical itself. The classic early experiments in which a mouse was submerged in a beaker of pre-oxygenated PFC emulsion and shown to breathe liquid continues to fascinate medical journalists and catch the public eye [1]. Similarly, the exchange-transfused "bloodless rat" experiments seemed to promise a quick transition to a clinically useful oxygen transport drug [2]. However, early PFC formulations were impure, persisted for long periods in the reticulo-endothelial system, and proved unsuitable for clinical trials.

Broad application of PFC as RCS may be limited by their oxygen-loading and off-loading properties (Fig. 1). Unlike blood and haemoglobin constructs, PFC dissolve O_2 in a linear fashion related directly to the partial pressure of O2. What this means in practice is that these emulsions can carry a great deal of O2, but only if the patient inspires high concentrations of supplemental O2. Furthermore, the compounds may release much of the O2 as blood passes through less well-oxygenated environments and long before it reaches the most ischaemic tissues. The latter property, the need for refrigerated storage and the relatively short-circulating half-life have led some investigators to postulate that these chemicals will prove most suitable for hospitals.

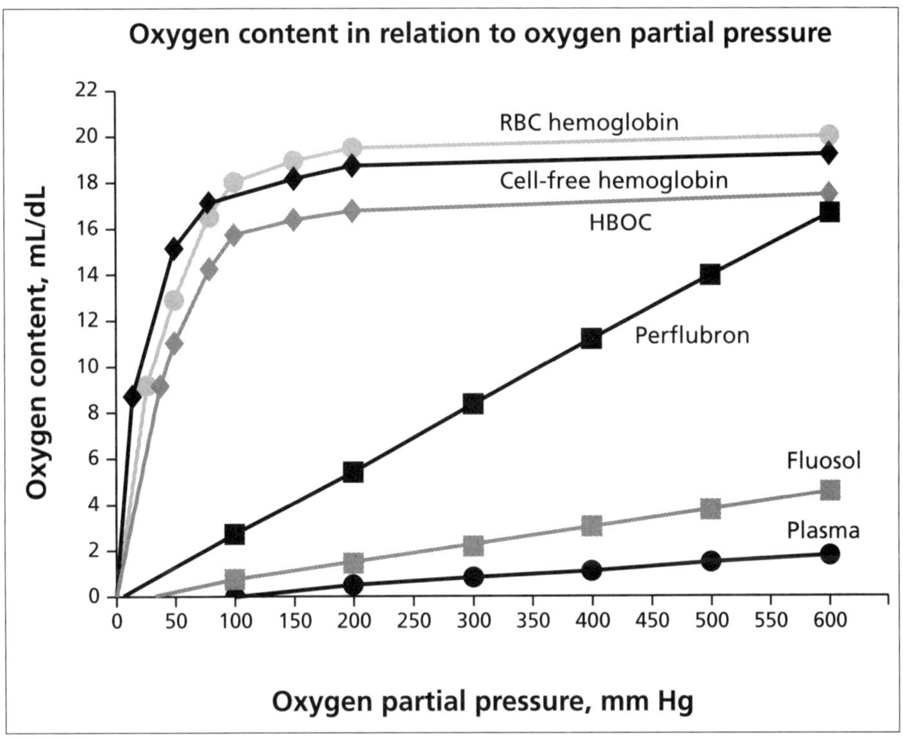

Fig. 1: Oxygen solubility/dissociation curves for blood (RBC haemoglobin), free haemoglobin, engineered HBOC and two perfluorochemical emulsions. Small changes in oxygen partial pressure in the ranges of low tissue pO_2, mixed venous pO_2 (40 mm Hg) and arterial pO_2 (100 mm Hg) result in large changes in the amount of O_2 bound or released. In contrast, perfluorochemicals dissolve O_2 in a linear fashion and require high pO_2 (supplemental O_2) to carry clinically relevant amounts of O_2.

During a 10-year period, thousands of patients with a wide variety of illnesses received an early PFC formulation, Fluosol DA. This agent was even licensed for use in coronary artery balloon angioplasty. However, in controlled clinical trials, patients receiving Fluosol failed to show substantial physiological benefit and were plagued with adverse reactions attributed by some to complement activation [3]. In any case, production of this drug ceased in 1994. An excellent review of this drug and other early PFC has been published by Keipert [4].

Newer PFC formulations are in phase III trials and a European multicentre, randomized study of orthopaedic surgery patients reported a reduced need for allogeneic blood during profound intra-operative haemodilution [5]. A study of general surgery patients is in progress. Troubling side effects associated with complement activation and cytokine release have been attenuated by newer formulations containing smaller emulsion particles. However, an influenza-like syndrome attributed to macrophage-mediated clearance of the emulsion, and a curious sequestration of 15-20 % of circulating platelets, are commonly observed. Phase III trials using PFC to augment profound perisurgical haemodilution have been suspended while an increased frequency of stroke in the treatment arm is investigated. It is not clear whether stroke was related to the PFC or to trial design, which included rapid, deep haemodilution at the onset of surgery. Despite the several questions that the trials in surgery have raised, the singular ability of these agents to dissolve gases, their ability to be sterilized, and their low cost and ease of manufacture continue to make PFC emulsions attractive not only as RCS, but also as oxygen-carrying therapeutic agents to treat stroke, myocardial ischaemia, sickle cell disease, and vascular occlusion, and as sensitizing agents for radiation and chaemotherapy of malignancy [6-11].

Haemoglobin-Based Oxygen Carriers (HBOC)

Ninety-eight percent of blood oxygen is carried by encapsulated haemoglobin, nature's oxygen transport protein. The well-known sigmoid shape of the oxygen dissociation curve describes how haemoglobin binds oxygen rapidly in the lung and releases it efficiently in the low oxygen environment of the tissues (Fig. 1). For these reasons, haemoglobin seemed the logical candidate for an RCS. However, mammalian evolution undoubtedly encapsulated haemoglobin for a reason. Outside the red cell, haemoglobin is vulnerable to oxidative inactivation and its chains dissociate into dimers that are cleared by and toxic to the kidney. Inside the red cell membrane the haemoglobin tetramer is stabilized, provided with organic phosphates that modify oxygen delivery, and protected from harmful oxidants.

Numerous HBOC have been created during the last quarter of a century and several have progressed to late clinical trials (Table 3). Most HBOC are derived from human or bovine blood washed to remove cellular debris, pasteurized, filtered, and passed over chromatographic columns to ensure purity. The tetramer is then chemically modified by any of a bewildering variety of methods to provide molecules of different size, molecular weight, oxygen affinity, viscosity, and oncotic activity. Recombinant haemoglobin molecules with features not found in nature have also been prepared. RCS can thus be customized for their intended use, provided that the characteristics necessary for that use are well defined. Most candidate HBOC have been engineered to mimic the characteristics of the whole blood oxygen dissociation curve and the solutions have frequently been prepared to mimic many of the characteristics of blood, albeit at a lower haemoglobin concentration. However, as with PFC emulsions, the physiology of O_2 delivery by small molecules that extravasate beyond the microcirculation is incompletely understood and it is possible that different affinity, viscosity, and oncotic pressure may eventually prove superior. Finally, in an ironic recapitulation of red cell evolution, haemoglobin has been encapsulated in liposomes to prolong its intravascular circulation. However liposomal haemoglobin has yet to realize the success of other liposome encapsulated pharmaceuticals and will not be further discussed in this summary.

Table 3: Status of major candidate oxygen carriers.

Product	Derivation	Trial	Indication
Polyheme (Northfield Labs)	human hgb	phase III	trauma, surgery
Haemopure (Biopure)	bovine hgb	phase III	surgical haemodilution
Haemolink (Haemosol)	human hgb	suspended	surgery, haemodilution
Sangart	PEG-human hgb	phase I	surgical haemodilution
HemAssist (Baxter)	human hgb	terminated	haemorrhagic shock
Optro (Somatogen)	recombinant hgb	terminated	surgical haemodilution
Oxygent (Alliance)	perflubron	suspended	surgical haemodilution

It has been surprisingly difficult to demonstrate efficacy with the candidate HBOC. In a detailed report of a single patient, Mullon et al described a 21-year old woman with life-threatening auto-immune haemolytic anaemia treated with a polymerized bovine haemoglobin preparation after severe reactions to repeated incompatible transfusions, and her rapidly falling haematocrit left few options other than oxygen carriers devoid of red cell membrane antigens [12]. In this situation, proof of drug efficacy is still indirect, since the lower limits of haemoglobin that humans tolerate have not been defined [13]. However, the reversal of signs, symptoms, and electrocardiographic evidence of ischaemia in this symptomatic anaemic patient are compelling, as is the laboratory evidence of reduced end-organ ischaemia. In this instance it seems reasonable to conclude that the eleven HBOC infusions over a seven-day period helped to sustain this patient until her auto-immune process remitted.

Refractory auto-immune haemolytic anaemia illustrates an extremely limited indication for RCS. Most clinical trials use “blood sparing” or “blood avoidance” during surgery as primary study endpoints and these have been approved by the regulatory agency. For elective surgery, the potential exists to reduce an estimated five million units of perioperative red cells transfused annually in the United States. However, the short 12- to 48-hour half-life of these small molecules limits their blood-sparing use. Mathematical modelling suggests that benefits will be confined primarily to non-anaemic patients who undergo extreme haemodilution and sustain large perioperative blood losses [14]. The potential applications include an estimated 600,000 CABG surgery patients (in North America), 625,000 orthopaedic surgery patients, and 70,000 men undergoing radical prostatectomy. While the short half-life of current candidate RCS all but precludes their use for managing chronic anaemia, a "second generation" product with a longer intravascular survival might find substantial application for the estimated 40 % of patients with lung or ovarian cancer who develop chaemotherapy-induced anaemia.

Universally compatible, readily available RCS could revolutionize the treatment of haemorrhagic shock. Six-unit HBOC infusions have been given in place of red cells during acute blood loss in trauma and surgery and the same investigators have administered up to 20 units without apparent toxicity [15]. However, successful controlled trials of therapeutic efficacy have yet to be reported. No one knows how many trauma patients in shock outside the hospital would survive solely because an oxygen-carrying agent is added to their resuscitation solution. Even in combat settings where haemorrhage is the major cause of death, authorities estimate that no more than 20 % of military casualties are potentially salvageable [16]. Tissue oxygen deprivation is a well-documented factor in the pathophysiology of haemorrhagic shock, but the therapeutic role of oxygen carriers and the point at which transfusion becomes critical are not well understood.

A major impetus for developing safer alternatives to blood has faded as risk-benefit calculus of transfusions has changed for the better in the United States. Newer treatments now have to compete with a very safe and familiar product. The combination of volunteer blood, stringent donor eligibility criteria and sensitive testing, particularly the addition of direct assays for viral nucleic acid, has reduced the risk of transfusion-transmitted hepatitis to fewer than one case per 100,000 units transfused, and has virtually eliminated the risk of transfusion-associated HIV [17]. Other risks have declined in parallel. However a spate of emerging agents, West Nile virus, SARS virus, and monkey-pox virus, in addition to parasites such as T cruzi and malaria, emphasize the continued vulnerability of our blood supply. In addition, more than two-thirds of the developing world's nations do not have adequate blood [18]. An estimated 13 million blood donations globally are not tested for HIV and hepatitis viruses, primarily in developing countries where 80 % of the blood supply comes from paid or replacement donors and where the population infected is large. Blood availability is scarcely better. Twenty-five percent of maternal deaths from pregnancy-related causes are associated with loss of blood. Operational problems, infrastructure costs and cultural issues pose seemingly insurmountable hurdles to building modern blood delivery systems in the same regions. Inexpensive RCS, even those that fail to meet the rigorous safety standards applied to blood, would allow patients to receive treatments ordinarily requiring blood transfusion and could improve health dramatically in many developing countries. Whether such a practice, or even clinical trials of such products, is ethically acceptable, remains a subject of intense debate [19].

RCS still face formidable hurdles. The apparent lack of serious toxicity should not obscure the cautions that have slowed RCS licensing. Small molecules such as cell-free haemoglobin deliver oxygen in a fundamentally different way. A great deal has been learned, but the physiological consequences and compensatory mechanisms remain incompletely understood. Freely diffusing RCS-bound oxygen may be responsible for gastro-intestinal irritability, hypertension, and the recently well-publicized "excess deaths" in trauma patients that led to the termination of clinical trials and to the withdrawal of two HBOC formulations from further development [20]. Most HBOC formulations exhibit a "pressor effect" generally attributed to the ability of haemoglobin to scavenge the vasodilator, nitric oxide. However, recent experimental evidence implicates a second mechanism involving autoregulation of capillary blood flow [21,22]. Whether this pressor effect can be put to therapeutic use, for example in septic shock, or whether it must be eliminated because of the difficulty in controlling the response of different vascular beds, remains to be determined.

Economics will also influence RCS use. If emotion is set aside, expensive alternatives to red cells should be justified on the basis of increased safety and efficacy. High cost may not prohibit use in nations such as the United States, where zero-risk transfusion has become religion, but expensive alternatives will be totally out of reach for the developing countries that need them the most.

What does this mean for the oncology patient? The first generation of effective RCS is nearing licensing. These will be novel agents, not miracle drugs. This first generation has the potential to reduce the need for allogeneic blood in patients who require extensive surgical procedures. A second generation might address the issue of chronic anaemia during chemotherapy. However we should temper our expectations until we learn more about the advantages and limitations of these agents. Blood transfusion has a long history and most physicians are relatively familiar, if not comfortable, with its safety and efficacy profile, particularly the long-term toxicity. In this regard, RCS are an unknown quantity. RCS will not replace the need for red cells, but they should reduce or eliminate the need for blood for some patients, and permit treatment of others who currently cannot be transfused. If problems of cost and intravascular half-life can be solved, these drugs should save countless lives in the developing world.

References

1 Clark LC, Gollan R: Survival of mammals breathing organic liquids equilibrated with oxygen at atmospheric pressure. Science 1966; 152: 1755-1756.

2 Geyer RP, Monroe RG, Taylor K: Survival of rats perfused with a perfluorocarbon-detergent preparation, in Norman JV, Folkman J, Hardison LE Ridolf LE, Veith FJ (eds): Organ Perfusion and Preparation, New York, Appleton-Crofts, 1968, pp 85-95.

3 Teicher BA, Schwartz GN, Sotomayor EA, Robinson MF, Dupuis MP, Menon K. Oxygenation of tumors by a hemoglobin solution. J Cancer Res Clin Oncol 1993; 120: 85-90.

4 Gould SA, Rosen AL, Sehgal LR et al: Fluosol-DA as a red cell substitute in acute anemia. N Engl J Med 1986; 314: 218-221.

5 Keipert PE: Perfluorochemical emulsions: future alternatives to transfusion, in Chang TMS (ed): Principles, Methods, Products and Clinical Trials, Zurich, Karger, 1998, pp 127-156.

6 Spahn Dr, van Brempt R, Theilmeier G et al: Perflubron emulsion delays blood transfusions in orthopedic surgery. European Perflubron Emulsion Study Group. Anesthesiology 1999; 91: 1195-1208.

7 Sakas DE, Whitaker KW, Crowell RM et al: Perfluorocarbons: recent developments and implications for neurosurgery, J Neurosurg 1996; 85: 248-254.

8 Premaratne S, Harada RN, Chun P et al: Effects of perfluorocarbon exchange transfusion on reducing myocardial infarct size in a primate model of ischemia-reperfusion injury: A prospective, randomized study, Surgery 1995; 1127:670-676.

9 Horn E-P, Standl T, Wilhelm S et al: Bovine hemoglobin increases skeletal muscle oxygenation during 95 % artificial arterial stenosis. Surgery 1997; 121: 411-418.

10 Teicher BA, Holden SA, Ara G et al: Restoration of tumor oxygenation after cytotoxic therapy by a perflubron emulsion/carbogen breathing. Cancer J 1995; 1:43-48.

11 Kaul DK, Liu X, Nagel RL: Ameliorating effects of fluorocarbon emulsion on sickle red blood cell-induced obstruction in an ex vivo vasaculature, Blood 2001; 98: 3128-3131.

12 Mullon J, Giacoppe G, Clagett C, McCune D, Dillard T: Polymerized bovine hemoglobin transfusions in a patient with severe autoimmune hemolytic anemia. New Engl J Med 2000; 342: 1638-1643.

13 Weiskopf RB, Viele MK, Feiner J et al: Human cardiovascular and metabolic response to acute isovolemic anemia. JAMA 1998; 279 (3): 217-221.

14 Brecher ME, Goodnough LT, Monk T: The value of oxygen-carrying solutions in the operative setting, as determined by mathematical modeling. Transfusion 1999; 39: 396-402.

15 Gould SA, Moore EE, Hoyt DB et al: The first randomized trial of human polymerized hemoglobin in acute trauma and emergent surgery. J Am Coll Surg 1998; 187: 113-122.

16 Fluid Resuscitation. State of the science for treating combat casualties and civilian injuries. Pope A, French G, Longnecker DE (eds): Washington, National Academy Press, 1999.

17 Busch MP: Closing the windows on viral transmission by blood transfusion, in Stramer SL (ed): Blood Safety in the New Millennium, Bethesda, American Association of Blood Banks, 2001, pp 33-54.

18 Safe blood starts with me. World Health Organization and International Federation of Red Cross and Red Crescent Societies. Geneva 2000:12.

19 Varmus H, Satcher D: Ethical complexities of conducting research in developing countries. N Engl J Med 1997; 337: 1003-1005.

20 Sloan EP, Koenigsberg M, Gens D et al: Diaspirin cross-linked hemoglobin (DCLHb) in the treatment of severe traumatic hemorrhagic shock. A randomized controlled efficacy trial. JAMA 1999; 282: 1857-1864.

21 Winslow RM, Gonzales A, Gonzales ML, et al: Vascular resistance and the efficacy of red cell substitutes in a rat hemorrhage model. J Appl Physiol 1998; 85 (3) 993-1003.

22 Winslow RM: Current status of blood substitute research: towards a new paradigm. J Intern Med 2003; 253: 508-517.

Dr. H.G. Klein, Department of Transfusion Medicine, Warren G. Magnuson Clinical Center, National Institutes of Health, Bdg 10, Rm 1C-711, Bethesda, MD 20892, U.S.A.
E-mail: hk29h@nih.gov

Vyas GN, Williams AE (eds): Advances in Transfusion Safety.
Dev Biol (Basel). Basel, Karger, 2005, vol 120, p 53.

SESSION VI

Panel and Open Discussion

Moderator: *R.Y. Dodd*

Vyas GN, Williams AE (eds): Advances in Transfusion Safety.
Dev Biol (Basel). Basel, Karger, 2005, vol 120, pp 55-56.

Testing, Inactivation or Both?

Moderator: *R.Y. Dodd*

Panelists: *M.E. Brecher, E.L. Snyder, J. Chapman, H.G. Klein*

Panel proceedings summarized by *A.E. Williams*

Dr. Dodd posed the following question to the panel:

Consider whether, 10 years in the future, we will be using multiplex testing (such as gene-chip based tests), pathogen reduction, or both for assuring blood safety?

The discussants largely agreed that pathogen inactivation technology would probably be a technical reality in the future for blood components and blood-derived biologics of the future, just as it currently is for plasma derivatives. The panel also generally agreed that new inactivation processes would most probably be an additive, rather than replacement technology within the developed world for major infections such as hepatitis and HIV. This opinion was held based both on the public's demand for optimal safety as well as predicted conservatism on the part of regulatory bodies until the data in support of inactivation as the sole protection against all transfusion-transmitted infections were time-tested and compelling. Examples to support this prediction included the long-standing requirement for serological tests for syphilis, despite an absence of transfusion-transmitted cases over the past 40 years, and the persistent requirement for donor screening for a history of hepatitis despite highly advanced test systems for screening donated blood. The observation was made that major paradigm shifts in medicine typically were not driven as much by new technology as by the rule of self-determination; i.e. the local evolution of thought regarding acceptance of risk and cost.

Hope was expressed that effective inactivation technologies might afford a measure of much-needed relief from the pattern of new test implementation that seems to follow identification of any new transfusion-transmitted agent. The developed world has many more healthcare dollars to spend, and could most probably find ways to afford new inactivation technologies that bring added value. However, it was also noted that even in a resource-rich environment, increased prioritization of available health dollars is likely to be the way of the future. Advances in transfusion-associated technology, while largely attainable in developed countries to date, have already altered the very structure of the blood transfusion community, resulting in increased consolidation and monopolization of both blood collection and blood transfusing institutions.

Panel discussants agreed that the moderator's question had to be considered quite differently in the context of the developing world, where 81 % of the world's blood-using population resides and where only 40 % of world's blood supplies are available – many of them at a lower standard of safety. The panel felt that numerous economic, political and ethical hurdles would have to be overcome to implement either improved testing or pathogen inactivation successfully. Pathogen inactivation does appear to have the unique potential to offer major public health benefits in the health care systems of developing nations not only through improved safety, but also by increased supply. In many instances a large proportion of potential donors are positive by current screening tests and in combination with inactivation processes, a larger pool of donors may safely become eligible for donation.

The hurdles in reaching this goal in the developing world are substantial, however. The general scarcity of healthcare resources and of skilled medical staffing require that innovations newly introduced into developing countries must be simple and cheap, and produced locally wherever possible. Since technology growth in the developing world is often by leaps (e.g. use of cellular phones in areas where no telephone lines exist), new technologies often must serve as stand-alone systems. The observation was also made that if the cost of even an ideal inactivation system greatly exceeded that of currently available blood screening tests, implementation would simply not be feasible.

A major barrier to approval of inactivation technologies in the developed world is the possible toxicity of the treatment itself and the effect of any residual inactivation chemicals that might remain in a transfused blood unit. In developed countries, the risk : benefit assessment of these procedures must clear a high bar, given the current high index of transfusion safety. In developing countries where much of the blood supply is inherently less safe, the risk: benefit assessment may be entirely different, and higher levels of residual toxicity (or lower acceptable levels of inactivation) may be feasible from a public health standpoint. However, ethical considerations have a major role in determining the best level at which risk of any type should be acceptable and these considerations remain complex.

Several panelists mentioned that even in the absence of major new technology transfer, blood safety in the developing world must continue to improve with the provision of simple, basic resources. For example, the problem of bacterial contamination could be greatly improved in the absence of inactivation systems through training for sterile phlebotomy, better donor screening measures, and improved quality systems in general.

Vyas GN, Williams AE (eds): Advances in Transfusion Safety.
Dev Biol (Basel). Basel, Karger, 2005, vol 120, p 57.

SESSION VII

Issues in Donor Recruitment and Selection

Moderator: *A.E. Williams*

Vyas GN, Williams AE (eds): Advances in Transfusion Safety.
Dev Biol (Basel). Basel, Karger, 2005, vol 120, pp 59-65.

Donor Recruitment and Education

N. Mikkelsen

Secretary General of the IFBDO, c/o Bloddonorerne i Danmark, Frederiksberg, Denmark

To present a general view of donor recruitment and education is no easy task, as conditions vary considerably from country to country. There are very specific cultural aspects to blood donation, which vary because of tradition, religion, respect for the health system, marketing and economic incentives. I have taken as my point of departure the situation in **Europe**, where almost 20 million full blood donations are taken each year, most of it from voluntary, non-remunerated blood donors.

The amount of blood products used per capita varies in Europe, largely due to: (i) the quality of blood-products (and associated low risks connected with use); (ii) tradition, the cost of blood products; (iii) the continued availability of a sufficient number of donors, and (iv) the level of acceptance of blood donation and confidence in the transfusion system.

A number of scientific studies have already been published about donor motivation: Why do people want to donate? What are the fears which prohibit them from donating? These are works of philosophers, psychiatrists, marketing experts etc. and I do not intend to compete with these learned people. As I am a lawyer, you will have to accept my views as that of a **layman,** drawing on my findings from a number of countries as Secretary General of the International Federation of Blood Donor Organizations.

What Brings the Donor to the Blood Bank?

The donor must first and foremost feel that the **national blood system functions well** – to the best advantage of his countrymen, his family and himself. He should have 100 % **trust** in the safety of the **products** and in the **adequacy of supply** when human blood is needed. And he must feel that he is an important part of the national blood supply.

To convince him, he must be well informed. **Information** is the **key incentive** to a well functioning blood supply. A coherent information policy should be part of the media strategy of blood banks and donor-associations, and also in their everyday contact with donors.

Finally, there should be no waste, no unnecessary transfusions, and no scandals. The **reputation** of the blood services must be as high as possible. **Accreditation** or ISO-certification can be of good use to increase the respect for the blood system from ministers, the media and others. And **transparency** is essential. A well-functioning blood supply has nothing to hide, apart from respecting the anonymity between donors and patients.

Of course, all blood must be **tested**. What is the good of giving blood, if patients become ill from HIV, HBV, HCV or syphilis ? There must be full **traceability** from donor to patient, and any relevant **abnormal findings** should be reported to the donor.

So to bring the donor to the blood bank, much work has to be done. And it is necessary to have the full **cooperation of government, blood bank staff and volunteers.**

Basic Guidelines

If you want their confidence, donors should know that there are **strong ethical principles** governing your national blood system. We are, after all, dealing with a part of the human body, which should be given **special respect**. Blood has therapeutic value with properties that can only be developed by a human being.

I am a fervent believer in **anonymous, voluntary, non-remunerated blood donation**, as defined by the Council of Europe in Recommendation (95) 14: "*Donation is considered voluntary and non-remunerated, if the person gives blood, plasma or cellular components of his/her own free will and receives no payment for it, either in the form of cash, or kind which could be considered a substitute for money. This would include time off work other than that reasonably needed for the donation and travel. Small tokens, refreshments and reimbursement of direct travel costs are compatible with voluntary, non-remunerated donation..*

This definition – and much other good advice for your blood system – can be found in my "bible": **the "Guide to the preparation, use and quality assurance of blood components",** which the **Council of Europe** has recently published in its 9th edition.

The principle of voluntary, unpaid donation has been strongly supported by the European Parliament and the EU Council of Ministers in December 2002 in the new **EU Directive on blood safety**, and I expect that the European Union in the coming years will take a number of initiatives to supplement the good work of the Council of Europe, using their expertise - and cooperating with voluntary donor organizations in Europe.

National donor organizations should, in co-operation with national health authorities, establish the **necessary guidelines** for blood donation. It is part of a democratic society that an organization is allowed to protect **the legitimate interest of the blood-donors,** as donors are an essential part of the blood supply. The guidelines established should inter alia guarantee full **anonymity** of the data collected, and ensure that donors have **no** other **legal obligations** than to answer questions about their health to the best of their knowledge. The end-use of blood and blood products should be clearly indicated, and respect the statement by the EU in its new Directive, that: *"Modern blood transfusion practice has been founded on the principles of* ***voluntary donor services, anonymity*** *of both donor and recipient,* ***benevolence*** *of the donor, and the* ***absence of profit*** *on the part of* ***the establishments*** *involved in blood transfusion services".*

Blood is a **gift** from the donor to an unknown receiver, and it should never, in any of its components, be treated like a piece of merchandise, if you want your donors to come back return.

National Self-Sufficiency

The WHO has consistently from 1975 onwards recommended voluntary, non-remunerated blood donation, as well as and national self-sufficiency.

National self-sufficiency in blood-products is an important aim for ethical and for safety reasons:

(i) for **ethical reasons**, since a country should not exploit donors from countries which need blood themselves. Donors come back, if they can take pride in the fact, that they are able so sustain a healthy blood supply for their own society; (ii) for **safety reasons**, since rules for blood-donation can be nationally established and controlled to ensure high quality of blood and blood-products with the smallest possible risk for the transfer of infections.

As members of the WHO World Health Assembly, Ministers of Health have adopted these recommendations, and they have, accordingly, taken upon themselves to ensure that sufficient **public funds are made available to cover the needs for recruitment and retention** of non-remunerated donors. Non-remuneration does **not** mean that recruitment and retention can be achieved without expenses – quite the contrary.

I am surprised to see how governments are ready to spend unending amounts of money to improve formal blood-security, buying test equipment etc. But they very often totally forget that the recruitment and retention of donors cost **money**. You can only obtain optimal safety if you have an abundant supply of donors and, hence, of blood. **A large donor population** allows the blood collectors to select the donors critically. Good conditions for donor-deferral is the safest and cheapest way to obtain optimal security.

I believe that recruitment money is best administered by **voluntary organizations**, and that volunteers are cheaper than paid recruiters. But I am strongly adverse to direct payment to donors: It degrades the act of blood donation and appeals to those groups of the population which we least want to see as donors.

In my experience, the most efficient use of funds for recruitment and retention is paying a small **fee per donation** and a small **fee for each active donor** belonging **to the local donor – associations,** to cover their expenses. The fee per donation relates to the expenses connected with recruitment and retention, while the fee per donor should cover continuing information activity to all potential donors, whether they donate often or seldom. Of course there must be complete transparency in the use of association funds, with proper accounting etc.

Local Donor Organizations

Donor associations should correspond largely to the number of bleeding-facilities, normally at local hospitals. Their main **tasks** include **donor-recruitment**, contact with blood-bank staff, local press contacts, distribution of tokens, donor parties and other **donor-retaining** activities.

The local donor association could well be made up of representatives from other **local popular organizations,** such as the scouts, sports associations, professional organizations, company representatives, policemen, firemen's associations, Rotary, Lions, church-groups etc.

The local associations could be regrouped in regional committees and in a **national** organization. The national organization should negotiate a **detailed agreement about conditions for blood-donation** with the relevant government agency, which has responsibility for health care and hospitals, including blood-banks.

The local donor organizations should be represented democratically at a regional and national level, and sufficient administrative support should be available for the national and regional organizations and their decision-makers.

Insurance

As an important service to the donors, there must be **full insurance** for the blood-donors to cover expenditures arising from personal injuries to a donor before, during or after the donation. Should an injury occur, **personal contact** should be taken **IMMEDIATELY** from the blood bank to **assist the donor** with economical or physical problems arising from the injury, so that proper treatment can be initiated at the earliest possible date.

Good Quality and Efficiency in Blood Services

Blood donors are normally modest people - and they do not complain easily. But they do feel strongly about **quality** and **efficiency in the blood services**. The **reputation** of the blood system is everything: The donor should be **proud** of belonging to the blood supply system of his country. Scandals, shortages and dramatic appeals should be avoided, and the media should be used professionally.

The safety of the donor and the recipient is paramount, and the donor should be well informed of what happens, if an accident should occur, including insurance, practical help, medical treatment etc.

There must be no waste and minimal outdating, and self deferrals, autologous or directed donation and peer pressure should be avoided. Use the best equipment possible – but in accordance with local economical circumstances (no unnecessary luxury, please).

Donors can "smell" inefficiency, and waiting in long queues should be avoided at all cost (especially if an appointment has been made, which most donors want). Efficient service includes a friendly environment, donor-friendly opening hours, pleasant rooms and beds, and well-equipped waiting rooms – before and after donation. And it would help if taxi-pickups arrive in time, that opening hours were followed, that parking-spaces were reserved for the donors, that beverages and food were good and sufficient, that letters were sent to the right addresses with the correct data etc. Repeat, regular donors should be recognized – and especially when they expect special recognition (for 10, 25, 50, 75, 100 donations etc.). Directed press-coverage should be sought on such occasions to raise the self-esteem of the donors.

Donors expect to be serviced by trained, medical professionals, before, during and after donation, and the methodological medical check-up should be taken seriously.

Donors should be very well informed – leaflets, posters and questionnaires should be 100 % correct and have a professional look. E-mail and web-sites should be used for a quick up-date of information. Donors are thinking human beings and should be respected as such.

Visible Donor Associations

The donor organizations must also be efficient and visible, if they are to fulfil their mission in a world with fierce competition for media attention. **High public visibility** is a must, and the national donor organization must seem to be **competent, professional**, and **reliable,** with a modern approach, but still with respect for the independence and competence of the local donor associations.

The donor associations should continuously **update themselves** and present an attractive picture of the cause of blood donation, in particular to young people.

The national donor organization should have a **logo**, which anyone in the country identifies with the blood donors' associations, and which is registered and protected by law. The same goes for the name of the organization and, preferably, only one national organization should be registered in each country. The organization should **act offensively in the media** and have a journalist and a marketing coordinator to promote press-campaigns, write leaflets and books for young people etc. Direct e-mail should be used to inform favourably inclined journalists and friends of the blood donors.

Telephone and **fax numbers** should be simple and easily remembered, and SMS and **e-mail services** and a **home page** should be established and **constantly updated** to remain attractive, not least to young people.

Newsletters, information leaflets and donor magazines should have a coordinated graphic expression and a **donor magazine should be mailed to all the donors** on a regular basis. Besides giving **relevant information** to the donors, they **pass it** to their children and friends. Sending the magazine by mail also **picks up any moves** – (and young donors especially tend to move around in their early years. But, most of all, the magazine gives the donors a feeling of **belonging to the blood supply ;** something they can be **proud** of and tell others about.

A **regular newsletter** – on paper and by e-mail – should be distributed at regular intervals to seek contact with friendly journalists to obtain positive and free media coverage of blood donation. Media catering for the young – television, youth magazines etc. – should also be contacted on a regular basis.

Once a year (for instance in connection with the World Donors' Day) a **national campaign** should be directed towards young people, with posters, free postcards etc., preferably based on a theme, which is also reflected in the donors' magazine. If possible, this could be supplemented by cinema spots or television spots, and advertisements in national newspapers and in youth magazines.

I can recommend **recruitment cards** being distributed at the exits from **ballot-places during election days** and at locals events, such a markets, local marathons, flying shows etc. **Rock-festivals** are also good for **the** distribution of information leaflets, recruitment cards etc.

This could be supplemented with **profile clothing** directed towards **young volunteers**, such as sweatshirts, polo-shirts, T-shirts, leather belts, donor caps and red umbrellas, all with the national blood donor **logo**. I can also recommend **telephone cards**, advertisements in **calendars** for young people, football books, study-books etc.

To receive more creative ideas I can recommend **poster competitions**, which give both publicity and many wonderful ideas for posters, stickers, front-pages and special leaflets addressed directly to young people etc.

National donor organizations should **work internationally,** participating actively in the International Federation. Many young people travel, speak foreign languages and feel engaged in international affairs – and they expect a modern donor association to do the same.

A major step would be to send active young volunteers to the **international youth forums** organized by the International Federation. Such gatherings are used for serious work and fun and, most importantly, to promote a feeling of togetherness in the task of promoting unpaid voluntary blood donation in the future. Between the youth forums there is a lively traffic on the Internet between these young people (18-30 years of age), which produces good exchanges of ideas, campaign materials etc.

I can strongly recommend that donor associations establish a group of **young ambassadors** who operate as informers about blood donation in **schools**, **festivals** and other places where young people meet. The young ambassadors should be trained before they are to meet other young people, and as direct spokespersons to other young people they can be most efficient in getting the message across.

Why Depend on Volunteers in Blood Donor Recruitment and Retention?

It is essential that **volunteers** are engaged in **the promotion of non-remunerated blood donation**. I simply fail to understand why many countries don't wish to "exploit" the very many resources volunteers can bring to donor recruitment and retention. Of course it can be troublesome for medical doctors, directors of blood banks and administrators of hospitals to deal with volunteers.

Volunteers have their own ways and, as they are unpaid, you have less control of them than of paid staff.

BUT

1. They very often have much larger **networks** than paid recruiters have, as they may belong to scout-groups, sports-organizations, trade-unions, Rotary, staff of large companies etc. etc.

2. They can **bring in fellow volunteers** – and individuals with a different prospect of society than medical doctors and hospital administrators.
3. Very often **paid recruiters** are **underpaid**, not least compared to the medical staff - and as the job is rather tedious, they **tend not to remain** for long in recruitment jobs.
4. Finally, you just can**not recruit** effectively **by telephone**. **You need** to be out there and have **personal contact**. For that you need many people (ambassadors), and very often the blood banks simply cannot afford to hire a sufficiently large number of people to ensure direct personal contact.

The easy way out is to **pay the donors**. But that is **not a good solution** for a number of reasons. Setting aside the safety issue (and who can discuss this better than I can), **paid donation gives the act of blood donation a LOW status**. Who respects a person who, for a small sum of money, will sell a part of his body? No-one, not even the blood-bank blood collectors, as I have seen in those countries which still permit paid donations.

It is essential for well functioning donor recruitment and retention that the act of **blood donation is respected**, and sometimes even praised by role models, queens and presidents.

All this is hard **work**. It is my firm impression, however, that the **EFFICIENT WORK** of **blood bank staff** and of **volunteer associations** and **their close cooperation** is the **key to success** in the continued recruitment and retention of a sufficient number of voluntary non-remunerated blood donors.

Dr. N. Mikkelsen, Secretary General of the IFBDO, c/o Bloddonorerne i Danmark, Vesterbrogade 191, DK-1800 Frederiksberg, Denmark.
E-mail: mikkelsen@bloddonor.dk

Vyas GN, Williams AE (eds): Advances in Transfusion Safety.
Dev Biol (Basel). Basel, Karger, 2005, vol 120, pp 67-75.

Initiatives to Improve Blood Donor Screening

S. Kleinman[1], *L. Katz*[2]

[1] Professor of Clinical Pathology, University of British Columbia, Vancouver, BC, Canada

[2] Vice President, Medical Affairs, Mississippi Valley Regional Blood Center, Davenport, IA, U.S.A.

Key words: Blood donor, blood safety

Historically, the pre-donation questionnaire (interview) has contributed to blood safety, especially in the era before laboratory testing for hepatitis and HIV. However, over the past 20 years, donor interview questions have increased in number, become more medically sophisticated, and have become more probing of socially sensitive behaviours. (i.e. sexual activities, injection drug use history). Although these questions have been added with the intent of deferring potentially infectious donors, the questions have not been validated for sensitivity or specificity, which would be an extremely difficult task given the low rate of infections in the prospective donor population [1].

Asking more questions does not necessarily equate with receiving correct answers to those questions that directly affect risks to recipients. Postulated reasons for the inability to obtain accurate answers include: (i) failure of the donor either to understand the content or significance of the questions (ii) the donor's psychological denial of risk; (iii) the donor's unwillingness to reveal socially sensitive behaviour to an interviewer or (iv) to leave the donation site without donating and (v) the inability of the donor to recall past events accurately (i.e. sexual behaviour from more than 20 years ago) [1-3]. Some of these factors may relate to poorly designed individual questions, others to a poorly designed questionnaire document, and still others due to psychological traits of the donor.

Data indicate that socially-sensitive donor interview questions do not always generate accurate responses. In 1993, using an anonymous post-donation mail survey, REDS investigators found that 1.9 % of respondents reported at least one behavioral risk that should have resulted in donor deferral [4]. Consistent findings were obtained with a second similar anonymous survey conducted in 1998 [5].

CURRENT QUESTIONNAIRES

Currently, in the U.S., each blood collection organization uses its own donor questionnaire. Problems with the current donor questionnaires include: (i) the large number of questions; (ii) the use of compound and multi-item questions (formatted in this fashion to allow the questionnaire to fit on one printed page, rather than to facilitate donor comprehension); (iii) the use of medical jargon with terminology that may not be understood by prospective donors (e.g. CJD, babesiosis) and (iv) the presentation of the questions in non-chronological order.

Previous attempts at standardization of the donor questionnaire in the U.S.

The first attempt at the standardization of donor questioning in different blood centres in the United States was by a consortium of California blood centres in the late 1980s [6]. The process used was one of consensus building among the medical directors of the various participating blood centres with the final questions approved by FDA. The limitations of this effort were the lack of pre-testing (i.e. validating) the questions in donor populations and the reliance on physicians rather than behavioral scientists to design the questions. In the 1990s, the American Association of Blood Banks (AABB) developed a Uniform Donor History Questionnaire (UDHQ) that has been pre-approved by FDA for use by any blood collection centre in the United States, provided that it is used without any alteration [7]. As new FDA recommendations for donor screening have occurred, the UDHQ has been continuously updated to reflect these changes. While many blood centres use portions of this questionnaire for donor screening, few currently use the fully intact version.

Previous attempts at validating donor questions

There is a need to validate the content of any donor-screening questionnaire to ensure that each question is fully understood across all demographic and educational strata of blood donors. Very little work had been done on validating or piloting donor questions until a recent study conducted by the American Red Cross. Seven donor interview questions were presented to six small focus groups composed of non-donors and facilitated by an educator and a blood services professional [8]. These questions were selected either because they frequently resulted in post-donation information from the donor which contradicted the response given at the time of donation or because the question focused on a rare disease (e.g. babesiosis, Chagas disease, Creutzfeldt-Jacob Disease). The results of the study suggested that the wording of several questions was sub-optimal and that rewording of the questions could improve donor comprehension.

REDESIGNING THE DONOR QUESTIONNAIRE AND RELATED MATERIALS

The multi-organizational UDHQ task force

At the request of FDA, a multi-organizational task force (including blood bankers, survey design experts, CDC and FDA staff) was convened under the auspices of AABB in mid-2000 to redesign a standardized UDHQ. The starting point for this activity was the then current AABB UDHQ. The primary aim of the project was to design a questionnaire that would maximize comprehension by donors; one limitation was that no FDA required or recommended questions could be removed. Several additional tasks were also taken on by the task force: these included rewriting pre-donation educational materials, developing an abbreviated questionnaire for frequent donors, and developing detailed instructions in the format of a User Brochure for use of these new materials by blood centre staff.

The redesign project

The process of questionnaire redesign included the use of two research methodologies (focus groups and cognitive evaluation) to validate that questions could be understood by the prospective donor population. The specific iterative redesign process included a detailed re-examination of each question by the task force with rewording, if necessary; presenting these questions to focus groups for feedback, further revision of selected questions based on focus group feedback, and performance of a cognitive evaluation of the entire questionnaire leading to final wording changes.

As part of this project, four focus groups were conducted under the auspices of the American Red Cross. The groups included both donors and eligible non-donors and included a spectrum of ages, gender, educational level, and ethnic backgrounds. The groups were presented with selected questions and asked for feedback, which in some cases, led to rewording of the questions. A cognitive evaluation of all potential questions on the UDHQ was then conducted by the National Center for Health Statistics under funding from the National Heart Lung and Blood Institute. One-to-one probing interviews were conducted in a laboratory setting by four trained interviewers with 35 participants recruited through advertising. The interviews were summarized into a written analysis that addressed the clarity and comprehensibility of each question. In addition to the UDHQ, the cognitive interviews also evaluated understanding of the medication deferral list and the pre-donation educational materials (see below). The final step in the redesign process was modification of selected questions by the task force based on cognitive interview results.

The redesigned UDHQ (currently under FDA review, see below) is presented in Figure 1.

	Yes	No	
Are you			
1. Feeling healthy and well today?	❑	❑	
2. Currently taking an antibiotic?	❑	❑	
3. Currently taking any other medication for an infection?	❑	❑	
Please read the Medication Deferral List.			
4. Are you now taking or have you ever taken any medications on the Medication Deferral List?	❑	❑	
5. Have you read the educational materials and had your questions answered?	❑	❑	
In the past **48 hours**			
6. Have you taken aspirin or anything that has aspirin in it?	❑	❑	
In the past **6 weeks**			
7. Female donors: Have you been pregnant or are you pregnant now? (Males: check "I am male.")	❑	❑	❑ I am male

	Yes	No	
In the past **8 weeks have you**			
8. Donated blood, platelets or plasma?	❑	❑	
9. Had any vaccinations or other shots?	❑	❑	
10. Had close contact with the smallpox vaccination site of someone else?	❑	❑	
In the past **16 weeks**			
11. Have you donated a double unit of red cells using an apheresis machine?	❑	❑	
In the past **12 months have you**			
12. Had a blood transfusion?	❑	❑	
13. Had a transplant such as organ, tissue, or bone marrow?	❑	❑	
14. Had a graft such as bone or skin?	❑	❑	
15. Come into contact with someone else's blood?	❑	❑	
16. Had an accidental needle-stick?	❑	❑	
17. Had sexual contact with anyone who has HIV/AIDS or has had a positive test for the HIV/AIDS virus?	❑	❑	
18. Had sexual contact with a prostitute or anyone else who takes money or drugs or other payment for sex?	❑	❑	
19. Had sexual contact with anyone who has ever used needles to take drugs or steroids, or anything <u>not</u> prescribed by their doctor?	❑	❑	
20. Had sexual contact with anyone who has hemophilia or has used clotting factor concentrates?	❑	❑	
21. Female donors: Had sexual contact with a male who has ever had sexual contact with another male? (Males: check "I am male.")	❑	❑	❑ I am male
22. Had sexual contact with a person who has hepatitis?	❑	❑	
23. Lived with a person who has hepatitis?	❑	❑	
24. Had a tattoo?	❑	❑	
25. Had ear or body piercing?	❑	❑	
26. Had or been treated for syphilis or gonorrhea?	❑	❑	
27. Been in juvenile detention, lockup, jail, or prison for more than 72 hours?	❑	❑	
In the past **three years** have you			
28. Been outside the United States or Canada?	❑	❑	
From **1980 through 1996**,			
29. Did you spend time that adds up to three (3) months or more in the United Kingdom? (Review list of countries in the UK)	❑	❑	
30. Were you a member of the U.S. military, a civilian military employee, or a dependent of a member of the U.S. military?	❑	❑	
From **1980 to the present**, did you			
31. Spend time that adds up to five (5) years or more in Europe? (Review list of countries in Europe.)	❑	❑	
32. Receive a blood transfusion in the United Kingdom? (Review list of countries in the UK.)	❑	❑	
From **1977 to the present**, have you			
33. Received money, drugs, or other payment for sex?	❑	❑	
34. Male donors: had sexual contact with another male, even once? (Females: check "I am female.")	❑	❑	❑ I am female
Have you **EVER**			
35. Had a positive test for the HIV/AIDS virus?	❑	❑	

	Yes	No	
36. Used needles to take drugs, steroids or anything not prescribed by your doctor?	❑	❑	
37. Used clotting factor concentrates?	❑	❑	
38. Had hepatitis?	❑	❑	
39. Had malaria?	❑	❑	
40. Had Chagas' disease?	❑	❑	
41. Had babesiosis?	❑	❑	
42. Received a dura mater (or brain covering) graft?	❑	❑	
43. Had any type of cancer, including leukemia?	❑	❑	
44. Had any problems with your heart or lungs?	❑	❑	
45. Had a bleeding condition or a blood disease?	❑	❑	
46. Had sexual contact with anyone who was born in or lived in Africa?	❑	❑	
47. Been in Africa?	❑	❑	
48. Have any of your relatives had Creutzfeldt-Jakob disease?	❑	❑	

Fig. 1: Proposed full-length questionnaire (UDHQ) as revised by the multi-organizational task force (under FDA review as of July 2003).

Several survey design principles have guided its development. In general, multi-part questions were divided into two or more narrowly focused questions. Questions were formulated using a time-bound approach (e.g. in the past x months, have you... ?). The entire questionnaire was formatted by grouping questions in chronological order from the most recent (e.g. in the past 48 hours) to the most remote (e.g. from 1977 to the present,... or: Have you ever). This strategy reduces the need for the donor to skip mentally from one time interval to another when answering the questions.

Based on the advice of survey design experts, the UDHQ was designed to be self-administered by the donor and the document was validated through cognitive interviewing using this approach. Self-administration consists of the donor reading each question and checking off yes or no answers on the donor card; unacceptable answers are reviewed and investigated further by an interviewer. In a recent guidance document, the FDA has stated that this method of questionnaire administration can be used for all donors [9].

The UDHQ retains the use of capture questions which are currently part of most donor interview questionnaires. An example of such a question is "In the past three years, have you been outside the U.S. or Canada?" A positive answer to such a capture question then requires further detailed questioning to determine donor eligibility.

The task force developed a new approach to asking questions about specific medications that require donor deferral. This approach lists such medications on a separate document known as the Medication Deferral List which is provided to each donor. A question on the UDHQ asks: "Are you now taking or have you ever taken any medications on the Medication Deferral List?" and the donor is referred to this document. This approach has several advantages: (i) it reduces the amount of text on the donor card; (ii) it allows space for a brief explanation of the reasons for deferral if a donor is taking one of these medications and (iii) it easily accommodates changes to the list without having to reprint the donor cards. The latter circumstance occurs periodically when new drugs with a teratogenic potential are licensed, thereby necessitating a deferral of the prospective donor for a temporary or indefinite time, depending upon the half-life of the medication.

The task force has also revised the pre-donation educational materials based on feedback from the focus group and cognitive interviews. The most significant change is a section that provides a definition of sexual contact as the phrase is used in various questions on the UDHQ. Simple straightforward descriptions are given for vaginal, oro-genital, and anal sex. Other basic features of the new materials are: (i) an emphasis on the need for prospective donors to give accurate and honest answers to the donor screening questions to ensure recipient safety and (ii) to encourage the prospective donor to ask questions of the donor centre staff if he/she does not understand any of the UDHQ questions.

To aid blood centre staff in administering the UDHQ, a user brochure has been prepared. The goal of this brochure is to provide details of how the questionnaire should be administered by including flow charts that determine donor eligibility and by indicating follow-up actions when positive answers to capture questions are obtained. The user brochure is not intended, however, to serve as a standard operating procedure (SOP); rather it is intended to be used in conjunction with each blood centre's SOP for determining donor eligibility.

A continual complaint of repeat donors has been the need to answer the same questions about events from the remote past at every donation. This lengthens the donation interview process which is frustrating to many repeat donors. Because of this, the task force has developed an abbreviated questionnaire for frequent donors. This abbreviated questionnaire retains questions about risk behaviours or changes in health status that might have altered since the donor's last donation, while eliminating questions about activities that could only have occurred in the remote. Donors will be eligible to use the abbreviated questionnaire if they have previously made two or more donations that have been screened with the full-length questionnaire, with at least one of these donations occurring in the previous six months. The rationale for this approach is that donors will have answered questions about the remote past on two occasions, thereby having been given a second independent opportunity to recall these events before the questions are no longer asked. The requirement for the previous donation occurring in the previous six months is so that a donor can focus on a short period for an evaluation of changes in risk or health. A challenge for blood centres desiring to use the abbreviated questionnaire will be to develop systems to ensure that it is administered only to those donors who meet the appropriate criteria.

Current and future status of the project

The materials designed by the task force have been submitted to FDA and have gone through several revisions in response to comments by FDA reviewers. At the time of writing, the review process is still in progress. Once approved, it is anticipated that the FDA will issue these materials along with a guidance document that addresses their use.

Since the beginning of the redesign project, several new potential threats to blood safety have arisen. FDA guidance documents relating to donor questioning and deferral with regard to smallpox vaccination, possible SARS exposure, and West Nile Virus symptoms have been issued for rapid or immediate implementation [10-12]. Because of the short time for the introduction of these questions, the FDA's suggested wording of the questions has not undergone the validation process that has been described above for the UDHQ. Although the need for rapid implementation may make it impossible to validate newly introduced questions before their use, a mechanism has recently been developed for retrospectively validating the clarity of such questions. The process will involve using cognitive interviewing by the National Center for Health Statistics as described above. It is expected that after such cognitive interviews are conducted, the results of the evaluation will be used to revise the wording of any newly introduced question that has been determined to be unclear.

Problems that may persist despite the redesign of the UDHQ

Despite the redesign of the donor questionnaire, inherent problems (such as (i) donor perception of lack of privacy; (ii) literacy level of the donor; (iii) limited English fluency; (iv) interviewer variation; (v) willingness of the donor to share sensitive information with another individual and (vi) the ability of the blood centre to revise the printed material quickly) will remain as long as the donor screening process and donor questionnaire are based on printed materials [1,2,13]. The only practical approach to the donor interview that can address these problems satisfactorily is the use of a computer-assisted (interactive) self-interview.

The Computer-Assisted Self-Interview (CASI)

The Computer-Assisted Self-Interview (CASI) can occur in several formats. The basic process can be enhanced by the use of: (i) an audio component (through headphones); (ii) a visual component (through illustrative graphics) and (iii) a touch screen format, which makes the process more user-friendly [9,14].

CASI with a sound component (audio-CASI) is now a preferred method of collecting information about sensitive behaviours such as sexual experience and illegal drug use. A recent study compared audio CASI with a self-administered questionnaire in a national survey of adolescents and found that the prevalence of behaviours such as male-to-male sex, injection drug use, and sex with an intravenous drug user was three-fold higher when audio-CASI was used [15]. Although the study was not entirely analogous to the blood donation interview in that no permanent record linked to the respondents identity was produced, these findings are nevertheless suggestive that CASI might enhance the truthfulness of responses to socially sensitive questions in the donor interview.

Advantages of CASI are numerous. It provides a sense of confidentiality and privacy since there is not a person-to-person interface. There is the potential for administration in multiple languages, with the language preference selected by the interviewee. Since computer administration obviates the need for the questionnaire to fit on one printed page, the need for multipart questions that violate survey design principles is eliminated. In addition, there is no need to use smaller print fonts or to reprint forms every time a new question is added.

Error rates in completion of the questionnaire should also be reduced for several reasons. Subjects have only a narrow range of data entry options, missed questions can be monitored and called to the donor's attention, and responses can be subjected to extensive internal validity checks before the final paper or electronic data record is produced.

There are further advantages to CASI with an audio component. Probably the most significant is that the ability to hear questions overcomes the barriers of illiteracy or inattention. All questions are asked using a standardized presentation by a single pre-recorded interviewer. The pace can be standardized or the interviewee can vary the speed of interview administration to suit his or her individual comfort.

The use of audiovisual, touch screen-CASI in blood donor screening has been demonstrated by the recent experience of the Mississippi Valley Regional Blood Center (MVRBC) in Davenport, Iowa [14]. This centre has used an audio-visual touch screen CASI (Quality Donor System ", Talisman, Inc.) to screen more than 50,000 donations at fixed collection sites over a two-year period. After the donor completes the CASI, the record is reviewed on-line by a trained donor screener who follows up all aberrant responses, annotates them, makes the decision as to donor eligibility according to standard operating procedures, and prints the final donor history form as a permanent record.

MVRBC has monitored a number of performance measurements since the implementation of CASI. First time donor deferral rates for HIV and STD related questions have significantly increased statistically compared to pre-CASI interviewing ($p = 0.017$; OR = 9.15, 95 % CI: 1.3 - 183.8). Error rates in completing the donor questionnaire have shown a statistically significantly decrease (> 60% decrease). In addition, the process has met with high levels of donor and staff acceptance on dimensions of privacy, time satisfaction, clarity and probable truthfulness.

In summary, this preliminary experience with audio-visual touch screen CASI at a single U.S. blood centre suggests that behavioral risks may be more accurately elicited and that error rates will decrease.

Conclusions

The efforts of the multi-organizational task force in redesigning the UDHQ should contribute to producing a donor-screening tool that is clearer and more comprehensible to prospective donors. Hopefully this will achieve the aim of obtaining more accurate answers to questions that defer donors who are at risk for transmitting infections to recipients. Further enhancements to donor screening will be achieved when CASI is more widely used.

Acknowledgements

I would like to thank Drs. Joy Fridey and Mary Townsend, the former and current chairs of the UDHQ multi-organizational task force, for providing resource material on the UDHQ resign project and for their efforts in moving the process forward.

References

1 Kleinman S, Williams AE: Donor selection procedures: is it possible to improve them? Trans Med Rev 1998; 12: 288-302.

2 Doll LS, Petersen LR, White CR et al: Human immunodeficiency virus type 1-infected blood donors: behavioral characteristics and reasons for donation. Transfusion 1991; 31: 704-709.

3 Mosley JW: Who should be our blood donors? (Editorial) Transfusion 1991; 31: 684-685.

4 Williams AE, Thomson RA, Schreiber GB et al: Estimates of infectious disease risk factors in US blood donors. JAMA 1997; 277: 967-972FDA.

5 Glynn SA, Smith JW, Schreiber GB, Kleinman SH et al: Repeat whole-blood and plateletapheresis donors: unreported deferrable risks, reactive screening tests, and response to incentive programs. Transfusion 2001; 41: 736-743.

6 Kolins J, Silvergleid AJ: Creating a uniform donor medical history questionnaire. Transfusion 1991; 31: 349-354.

7 American Association of Blood Banks: Uniform donor history questionnaire. Association Bulletin #95-5, June 2, 1995; access at www.aabb.org.

8 Orton SL, Virvos VJ, Williams AE: Validation of selected donor screening questions: structure, content, and comprehension. Transfusion 2000; 40: 1407-1413.

9 FDA. Guidance for Industry: Streamlining the donor interview process: recommendations for self-administered questionnaires. July 2003.

10 FDA: Guidance for Industry: Recommendations for deferral of donors and quarantine and retrieval of blood and blood products in recent recipients of smallpox vaccine (Vaccinia virus) and certain contacts of smallpox vaccine recipients. Final Guidance December 2002.

11 FDA: Guidance for Industry: Recommendations for the assessment of donor suitability and blood product safety in cases of suspected severe acute respiratory syndrome (SARS) or exposure to SARS. Final Guidance April 2003.

12 FDA: Guidance for Industry: Revised recommendations for the assessment of donor suitability and blood and blood product safety in cases of known or suspected West Nile Virus infection. Final Guidance May 2003.

13 Kline L, Friedman LI, Dempesy D et al: Assessment of blood donor privacy during health history interviews. Transfusion 1996; 36: 456-459.

14 Katz L, Rogenski L, Cumming P. Touch Screen, audio visual-computer assisted self interview (AV-CASI): First year results. (Abstract) Transfusion 2002; 42Supp: 114S.

15 Turner CF, Ku L, Rogers SM, et al: Adolescent sexual behavior, drug use, and violence: increased reporting with computer survey technology. Science 1998; 280: 867-873.

Dr. S. Kleinman, 1281 Rockcrest Avenue, Victoria, BC, V9A-4W4, Canada.
E-mail: skleinman@shaw.ca

Vyas GN, Williams AE (eds): Advances in Transfusion Safety.
Dev Biol (Basel). Basel, Karger, 2005, vol 120, pp 77-82.

Iron Balance in the Red Blood Cell Donor

G.M. Brittenham

Columbia University College of Physicians and Surgeons, New York, NY, USA

Key words: Iron, iron balance, iron supplementation, blood donor

Abstract: Phlebotomy of a unit of blood produces a loss of 200 to 250 mg of iron in haemoglobin. Because of physiological differences in iron balance between women of childbearing age and men, the loss of similar amounts of iron at donation has divergent consequences for committed donors. Women of childbearing age have an increased risk of iron deficiency if they donate more than one unit per year while men are usually able to maintain iron balance while donating four or more units of blood per year. Lack of iron is the most important medical reason for deferral from repeat donation and primarily affects women of childbearing age. Deferral of these women discourages them from further donation and may lead to their loss as donors. Provisions for blood donation should protect those who give blood from adverse consequences of their altruism. Safe and effective approaches to iron replacement after donation have been developed that can prevent iron deficiency in women who give blood repeatedly. Blood centres should consider incorporating programmes of iron replacement for women of childbearing age who give blood repeatedly to protect these donors against iron deficiency and to enhance their retention and commitment as dedicated donors.

INTRODUCTION

In the United States, the national blood supply depends upon the voluntary, repeated donations of a small minority of the population. Each donation of a unit of whole blood produces a loss of 200 to 250 mg of iron in haemoglobin. Because of physiological differences in iron balance between women of childbearing age and men, the loss of similar amounts of iron at donation has divergent consequences for committed donors. Men are usually able to maintain iron balance while donating four or more units of blood per year but women of childbearing age have an increased risk of iron deficiency if they donate more than one unit per year. After considering the effects of whole blood donation on iron balance in men and women, potential approaches to the prevention of iron deficiency in women of childbearing age who are committed donors will be described.

Iron Stores in Women and Men

The magnitude of differences in iron stores between males and females in the United States has recently been evaluated by a new approach that estimates body iron more precisely than had been possible with earlier techniques. This method, developed by Cook and colleagues [1], calculates body storage iron (expressed as milligrams storage iron per kilogram of body weight) for each individual examined by using the ratio of the concentration of serum transferrin receptor to that of serum ferritin. Body iron stores estimated with this method are shown in Figure 1 as a function of age for a sub-sample of participants in the third U.S. National Health and Nutrition Examination Survey (NHANES III). The results graphically summarize the effects of the iron demands of growth, menstruation and pregnancy on body reserves [2]. For both sexes, mean magnitudes of iron stores are almost identical until adolescence. In males, amounts then rapidly rise to a plateau in the third decade that is then followed by a gradual increase until the sixth decade when stores decrease slightly. In females, storage iron does not increase until the third decade because of the iron demands of menstruation and childbearing. Iron reserves then show little change until after the age of menopause; subsequently, stores progressively increase to reach levels near those in males by the seventh decade. Further analyses of these data [1] indicated that iron stores in U.S. men between 20 and 65 years of age had a single normal distribution, with a mean corresponding to about 752 mg of iron. In U.S. women between 20 and 45 years of age, two normal populations were identified, the larger (93 percent) with a mean corresponding to about

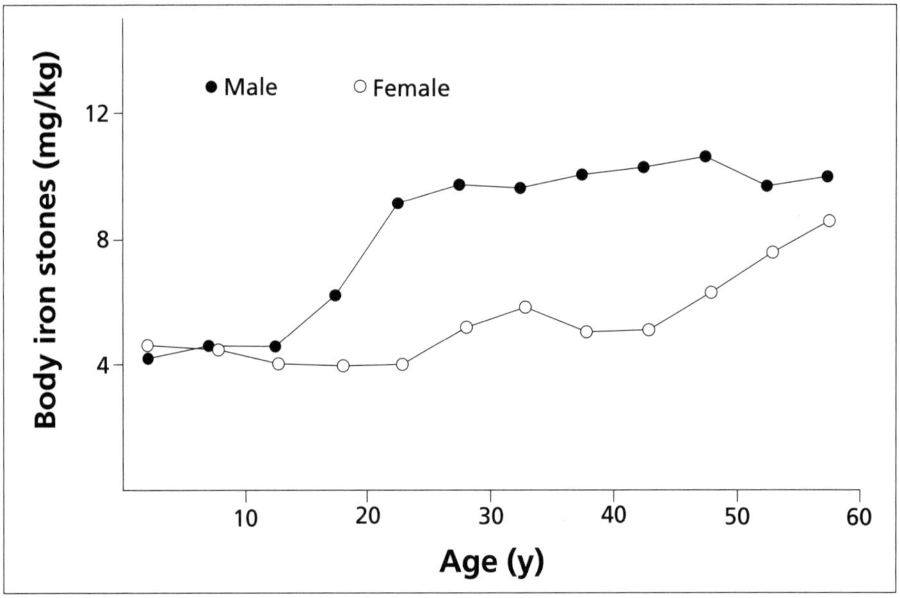

Fig. 1: Effect of age on body iron stores. All values for body iron are positive and indicate the amount of storage iron. Data are based on a convenience sample of 2057 samples collected in NHANES III. Shaded areas represent the mean ± 1 S.E.M. for each five-year interval. Reproduced from Cook [1], with permission.

297 mg of iron, and the smaller (7 percent) population with iron deficiency and absent iron stores [1]. Thus, in men, the mean magnitude of iron stores corresponds roughly to that in three units of blood. In women of childbearing age who are not iron-deficient, the average amount of the iron reserve is only slightly more than the iron content of a single unit of blood.

Effects of Blood Donation on Iron Balance in Women and Men

With an average amount of storage iron in a woman of childbearing age of only about 300 mg, the loss of 200 to 250 mg of iron with the donation of a unit of whole blood requires the subsequent mobilization of much or all of this reserve. If iron stores are not replaced, further donations of blood will produce iron deficiency and then anaemia. Normally, iron balance is maintained by controlling gastro-intestinal iron absorption [3]; iron stores and iron absorption are reciprocally related so that as stores decline absorption increases. In women who donate blood repeatedly, iron absorption from a usual diet cannot increase sufficiently to replace the iron losses from phlebotomy. Because of menstrual losses of iron, which average 13.5 mg per month, menstruating woman have a higher estimated daily iron requirement than men (1.5 vs. 1.0 mg) [4]. For both women and men, a minimum acceptable interval between donations of 56 days is recognized by the U.S. Food and Drug Administration (FDA) and national blood collection services. For menstruating women who donate at this interval, an iron loss of 200 mg at donation increases their estimated daily iron requirement to about 5 mg per day. Because the maximum iron absorption from a usual Western diet is at most 3 to 4 mg per day [2], a net deficit of 56 to 112 mg of iron would be expected in the 56 day interval. Repeated donations on this schedule make iron deficiency and then anaemia inevitable. By contrast, with larger initial iron stores, lower daily iron requirements and diets with greater amounts of bio-available iron, men are able to maintain iron balance while donating four or more units of blood per year [5]. Compared with men who have not given blood, male blood donors have decreased iron stores but in most some iron reserves remain and the absence of storage iron is uncommon. Consequently, current provisions for blood donation make a disproportionate iron demand on women of childbearing age [4].

These considerations of the effects of blood donation on iron balance in women of childbearing age are supported by studies of the prevalence of iron deficiency in committed donors. Practically every investigation of the iron status of women who give blood has confirmed that iron deficiency is a common problem and the major factor limiting the frequency of repeated donations [4-10]. Iron deficiency has been found in 18 to 50 percent of menstruating women *accepted* for repeat blood donation [5,6,9]. The prevalence of iron deficiency increases with an increasing frequency of blood donation per year rather than with the cumulative total of donations [5,6]. In one careful study, the prevalence of iron deficiency was 15 percent in women of childbearing age donating for the first time but increased to 30 to 48 percent in those making four to five donations per year without iron supplements [5].

Lack of iron is the most important medical reason for deferral from repeat donation and primarily affects women. One recent estimate is that deferrals due to low haemoglobin concentrations affect more than 700,000 prospective donors in the United States each year and that as many as 95 percent of those deferred are women of childbearing age [11]. Although deferral from donation for iron deficiency is short-term and temporary, the experience of deferral often has lasting consequences on the return of the donor for subsequent donations. For example, as many as 75 percent of donors deferred during a one-year period do not donate in the following year [11]. From their studies, Piliavin and Callero concluded that "a major factor in the loss of women from the donor pool may be depletion of iron stores, leading to deferral and subsequent discouragement from donation" [12].

Prevention of Iron Deficiency in Women of Childbearing Age who Are Committed Blood Donors

Provisions for blood donation should protect those who give blood from adverse consequences of their altruism. Three general approaches are available for the prevention of iron deficiency in women of childbearing age who are committed donors: further limitation of the frequency of blood donation, improved methods for detection and deferral of iron-deficient donors, and iron supplements. The first option, limiting donations by women of childbearing age to one to two units per year, would reduce their iron losses but is viewed unfavourably by many of the women who would be affected and would further decrease the national blood supply. The second option, attempting to exclude iron-deficient donors by changing screening procedures, seems impracticable. Increasing the haemoglobin concentration required for acceptability for donation is likely to be unacceptable. Only standards for haemoglobin concentration that would exclude most donors would protect against iron depletion [5]. Adding other means of detecting iron deficiency, such as measurements of the serum ferritin concentration, of the serum transferrin concentration, or of reticulocyte indices, would add cost and complexity to the screening, result in the deferral of more donors and would also reduce the national blood supply.

Iron supplementation, the third option, provides a potential means of preventing iron deficiency that was the subject of a recent workshop sponsored by the National Heart, Lung and Blood Institute [11]. Blood centres have been reluctant to supply routine iron supplementation because of (i) the possibility of masking underlying pathological conditions associated with blood loss; (ii) the risk of giving iron to individuals with undiagnosed hereditary haemochromatosis, and (iii) the risk of accidental iron poisoning in the small children of donors that is associated with the preparations of ferrous sulfphate and other iron salts. The workshop considered that an approach of using iron supplementation to prevent, not treat, iron-deficiency anaemia in women who are committed blood donors merited further consideration by blood centres. This programme, successfully applied in research studies [13,14], uses short-term administration of low-dose iron after giving blood to replace the iron that was lost at donation. No additional testing of donors is needed. To minimize the risks to donors with unrecognized pathological conditions associated with blood loss or with undiagnosed hereditary haemochromatosis, participation in the programme of iron replacement is restricted to women, 18 to 40 years of age, who are menstruating, committed to donating at least two units of blood each year, and have no personal or family history of hereditary haemochromatosis, intestinal polyps, colon cancer, or chronic gastro-intestinal or other medical disorders [11]. After each successful donation, eligible women would be offered 56 capsules, each containing 100 mg of carbonyl iron, and instructed to take one capsule at bedtime. After completing the 56-day course of iron replacement, each donor would again be eligible to donate. Subsequently, after each successful donation, the donor would receive another course of carbonyl iron replacement [11]. Carbonyl iron, a safe, non-toxic form of elemental iron that virtually eliminates the risk of iron poisoning [13,15], is suggested for the programme of iron replacement to minimize the risk of accidental poisoning in infants and children. Unit doses of preparations of ferrous iron or of other iron salts might also be used in such a programme with relative safety. The workshop concluded that the blood centres need to recognize the vulnerability of women of childbearing age to iron deficiency as a result of giving blood and to develop programmes to maintain iron balance in committed donors [11]. Prevention of iron deficiency is in the best interest of women who give blood and will help prevent their loss from the donor pool.

Conclusions

Women of childbearing age generally have lower iron stores, greater iron requirements and diets with less bio-available iron than men. Consequently, women have an increased risk of iron deficiency if they donate more than one unit per year while men can usually maintain iron balance while donating four or more units of blood per year. Among women of childbearing age who give two or more units of blood per year, iron deficiency is a common problem and the major factor limiting the frequency of repeated donation. Deferral of these women discourages them from further donation and may lead to their loss as donors. Safe and effective approaches to iron replacement after donation have been developed that can prevent iron deficiency in women who give blood repeatedly. Blood centres should consider the incorporation of programmes of iron replacement for women of childbearing age who give blood repeatedly to protect these donors against iron deficiency and to enhance their retention and commitment as dedicated donors.

Acknowledgements

This work was supported, in part, by research grants (R01 HL042439, R01 DK052709 and R01 DK066251) from the U.S. National Institutes of Health.

References

1 Cook JD, Flowers CH, Skikne BS: The quantitative assessment of body iron. Blood 2003; 101: 3359-3364.

2 Bothwell TH, Charlton RW, Cook JD, Finch CA: Iron Metabolism in Man. Oxford, Blackwell Scientific Pubications, 1979, pp 7-81.

3 Pietrangelo A: Physiology of iron transport and the haemochromatosis gene. Am J Physiol Gastrointest Liver Physiol 2002; 282: G403-G414.

4 Skikne B, Lynch S, Borek D, Cook J: Iron and blood donation. Clin Haematol 1984; 13: 271-287.

5 Simon TL, Garry PJ, Hooper EM: Iron stores in blood donors. J Am Med Assoc 1981; 245: 2038-2043.

6 Finch CA, Cook JD, Labbe RF, Culala M: Effect of blood donation on iron stores as evaluated by serum ferritin. Blood 1977; 50: 441-447.

7 Simon TL, Hunt WC, Garry PJ: Iron supplementation for menstruating female blood donors. Transfusion 1984; 24: 469-472.

8 Garry PJ, Koehler KM, Simon TL: Iron stores and iron absorption: effects of repeated blood donations. Am J Clin Nutr 1995; 62: 611-620.

9 Alvarez-Ossorio L, Kirchner H, Kluter H, Schlenke P: Low ferritin levels indicate the need for iron supplementation: strategy to minimize iron-depletion in regular blood donors. Transfus Med 2000; 10: 107-112.

10 Milman N, Byg KE, Ovesen L. Iron status in Danes 1994. II: Prevalence of iron deficiency and iron overload in 1319 Danish women aged 40-70 years. Influence of blood donation, alcohol intake and iron supplementation. Ann Hematol 2000; 79: 612-21.

11 Bianco C, Brittenham G, Gilcher RO, Gordeuk VR, Kushner JP, Sayers M, Chambers L, Counts RB, Aylesworth C, Nemo G, Alving B. Maintaining iron balance in women blood donors of childbearing age: summary of a workshop. Transfusion 2002; 42: 798-805.

12 Piliavin JA, Callero PL: Giving blood: the development of an altruistic identity. Baltimore, Johns Hopkins University Press, 1991, p 5.

13 Gordeuk VR, Brittenham GM, Bravo J, Hughes MA, Keating LJ: Prevention of iron deficiency with carbonyl iron in female blood donors. Transfusion 1990; 30: 239-245.

14 Brittenham GM, Gordeuk VR, Bravo JR, Hirschler NV, Piliavin JA, Goormastic M, Keating LJ: Carbonyl iron supplementation for female blood donors. Blood 1996; 88 (Suppl. 1): 360a.

15 Whittaker P, Ali SF, Imam SZ, Dunkel VC: Acute toxicity of carbonyl iron and sodium iron EDTA compared with ferrous sulfate in young rats. Regul Toxicol Pharmacol 2002; 36: 280-286.

Dr. G.M. Brittenham Columbia University College of Physicians and Surgeons, Harkness Pavilion, Room HP568, 630 West 168th Street, New York, NY 10032 USA.
E-mail: gmb31@columbia.edu

Vyas GN, Williams AE (eds): Advances in Transfusion Safety.
Dev Biol (Basel). Basel, Karger, 2005, vol 120, p 83.

SESSION VIII

Paid vs. Voluntary Plasma Donation

Moderator: *P.F. Strengers*

Vyas GN, Williams AE (eds): Advances in Transfusion Safety.
Dev Biol (Basel). Basel, Karger, 2005, vol 120, pp 85-96.

International Movement of Plasma and Plasma Contracting

A. Farrugia

Blood & Tissues Unit, Office of Devices, Blood and Tissues, Australian Therapeutic Goods Administration, Woden, Australia

Key words: Plasma, contract, standards, safety

Abstract: Plasma fractionation is a global business characterised by technological stability, increasing consolidation and a high level of regulatory oversight. All these factors affect the ease with which plasma derivatives can be accessed in the world market. As domestic regulatory measures in the first world blood economies become increasingly resonant to the precautionary approach, the availability of plasma as a raw material, as well as its cost, become an increasingly significant component in the cost of the final product. This decreases the amount of plasma which fractionators are able to allocate for export activities. Also, regulatory standards in the country of manufacture will reflect priorities in that country which may not be similar to those in export markets, but which will affect entry to those markets. While many countries possess a fractionation capacity, the limiting factor in supply worldwide is the amount of plasma available, and nationalistic drivers for each country to have its own plant are inimical to product safety and supply. Rather, the provision of sufficient supplies of domestic plasma should be the focus of resource allocation, with a choice of an appropriate contract fractionator. However, contract fractionation too may be affected by domestic considerations unrelated to the needs of the country of plasma origin. This chapter will review the global plasma market and the influences on plasma and plasma product movement across national borders. Problems in ensuring adequate safety and supply will be identified, and some tentative approaches to the amelioration of current barriers to the provision of plasma derivatives will be outlined.

INTRODUCTION

At some stage in the development of health care systems, the need for therapeutics derived from the large-scale fractionation of human plasma becomes felt. The stimulus for the manufacture of the first widely used plasma derivative – albumin solution – was the need for a stable blood volume replacement in battlefield casualties in the Second World War. After over fifty years of established use for this indication, its therapeutic validity was thrown into doubt following scrutiny of the available clinical safety data through a widely recognised meta-analysis process

[1]. This event stimulated the plasma fractionation industry to mount a vigorous and well financed rebuttal [2], but it still resulted in an apparent shift in clinical practice in several places, as reflected in a sharp decrease in albumin usage [3]. Concentrates of blood coagulation factors VIII and IX, for the past three decades a mainstay product for the industry, are rapidly being substituted with recombinant versions in the developed countries. While no apparent competitor to the other mainstay product – intravenous immunoglobulin – is currently apparent, and while the consumption of this product is still increasing, the pressures on the industry, to the extent of questions on its viability arising from the industry itself [4], are formidable. Despite this, the industry still supplies a worldwide market of $5.3 billion through the fractionation of 22 million litres of plasma [5] (Fig. 1). With many of the major fractionators drawing upon plasma supplies from collection centres in different countries, the ability to manufacture plasma collected from a range of environments is crucial if the supply of products is to be maintained. Similarly, the restriction of entry of finished products into national markets will necessarily affect supply.

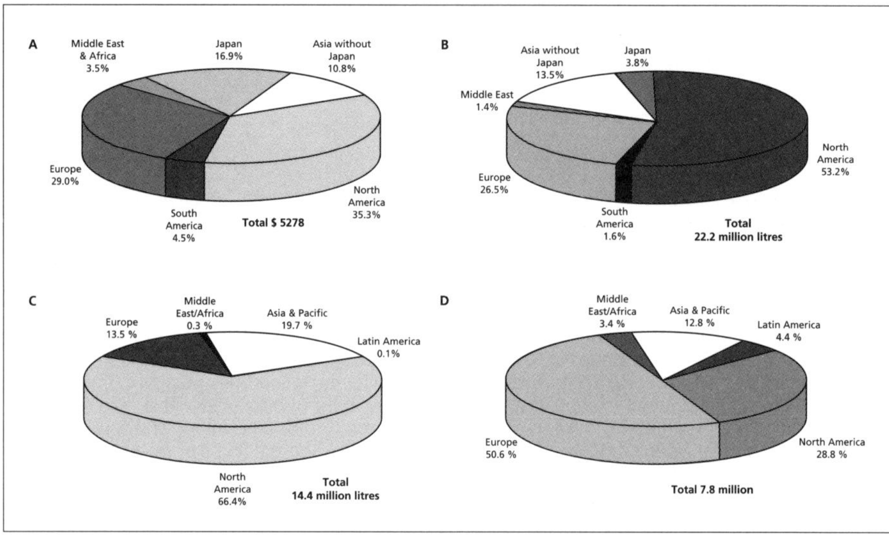

Fig. 1: Features of the plasma products industry.

A = Total market value
B = Total plasma collections
C = Source plasma collections
D = Recovered plasma collections

Courtesy: Market Research Bureau 2002

Factors Affecting Plasma Supply and Movement

Policy considerations

While twothirds of the current worldwide supply of fractionated plasma is generated through source (apheresis) plasma collection which is detached from the mainstream blood banking sector, the remainder is recovered as a by-product of whole blood collections in transfusion services supplying a range of products for hospital use [6], frequently integrated into national health care delivery systems. As these services develop to the stage where blood component therapy is feasible and clinically acceptable, a surplus of plasma relative to clinical transfusion needs may be expected and may be used for generating fractionated products. Under these circumstances, national policy makers are faced with the choice of generating a domestic fractionation capacity or of contracting with an external fractionation agency for the manufacture of their plasma into finished products. While the possession of a fractionation capacity is of advantage in some circumstances, it is doubtful if its generation de novo is a wise allocation of resources while these are needed for the infrastructure necessary for adequate plasma procurement. It appears from the available information [6] that current fractionation capacity worldwide is adequate and is not limiting the supply of products, while plasma supplies are still lagging behind needs in many countries. Therefore, continuing pressures to set up domestic fractionation plants for reasons other than objective needs are to be viewed with concern.

Opportunities to contract fractionation requirements on an appropriate regional basis are to be particularly encouraged. A particularly promising development in recent years has been the decision by the Brazilian authorities to construct a fractionation plant for national and possibly regional needs [7]. However, this particular example also demonstrates some of the problems encountered with this approach. While the possibility of regional fractionation has been offered by Brazil, the apparent intention of other Latin American countries to proceed with their own fractionation plants is to be viewed with some concern [8]. This is particularly the case when many such countries still lack adequate supplies of blood for their mainstream clinical needs, as judged relative to conventional norms. Another possible issue with the Brazilian project is the underestimation of actual needs. A 200-tonne capacity plant is envisaged, which for a population of 170 million is not commensurate with a realistic needs assessment; in Australia, a capacity of 250 tonnes caters for a population of 20 million. In this context, the Brazilian policy's stated aim of self-sufficiency contrasts with the projected supply of 20 % of national FVIII needs at 30^6 units, leading to an estimate of 0.9 IU/head of population as the final – inadequate – target level of FVIII supply to the haemophilia A community. It is thus important that worthy efforts such as the current example are underpinned by an adequate policy framework, including a realistic assessment of the country's plasma products needs and plasma generating capacity [9]. Such a framework may be structured around the considerations developed by the Global Collaboration for Blood Safety as outlined in Figures 2 and 3.

Issues around standards

Adequate oversight of international plasma movements is essential, if undesirable events such as the mysterious "Albovina" scandal are to be avoided [10]. The Australian Parliament's criticism of the national therapeutics regulator, when it perceived the latter's oversight of imported plasma activity as inadequate, illustrates the substantial pressures and expectations of the public and their elected representatives in sensitive issues such as plasma safety [11]. The oversight of plasma for fractionation includes standards that are necessary for assuring quality and safety in the final products, which are manufactured from the starting plasma. Currently, manufacturers operating on the international market have to conform to a number of standards, which are not always harmonised to a sufficient extent. Furthermore,

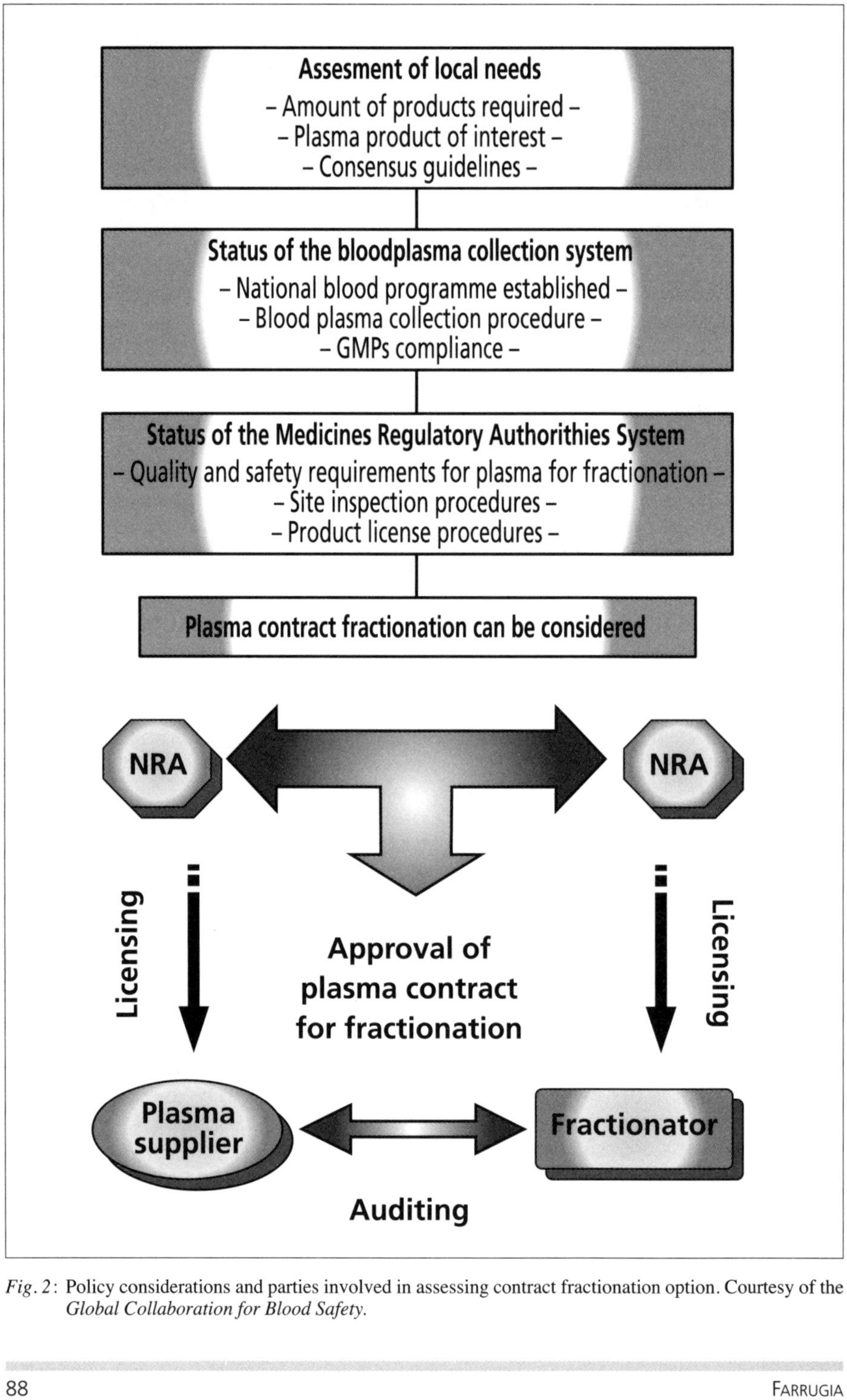

Fig. 2: Policy considerations and parties involved in assessing contract fractionation option. Courtesy of the *Global Collaboration for Blood Safety*.

differences between standards (Table 1) are not always scientifically justifiable. For example, the European Pharmacopeia (EP) requirement for serological re-testing of the plasma pool is difficult to justify in the era of NAT and robust viral inactivation. The EP's specification of FVIII levels cannot be related to the basic need for assuring the quality and safety of the plasma and such parameters are best restricted to arrangements between the manufacturer and the supplier. There is also a need to underpin freezing and storage requirements with basic scientific understanding. Statements justifying current requirements with vague allusions to the eutectic

Checklist – Prerequisites for supply of plasma for fractionation

- ❒ Features of plasma supply
  - ❍ Ensuring continuity of plasma supply
  - ❍ Origin: – whole blood and/or apheresis
- ❒ Safety & Quality
  - ❍ Donor selection
  - ❍ Testing
  - ❍ Epidemiology
  - ❍ Processing eg separation, freezing
  - ❍ Cold chain maintenance – storage, transport etc.
- ❒ Quality Systems
  - ❍ Auditing
  - ❍ Traceability
  - ❍ Good manufacturing practices (GMP's)

Economic considerations

- ❒ Collection cost of plasma, including donor recruitment
- ❒ Testing procedures on single donations
- ❒ Storage of plasma
- ❒ Transportation of plasma (by sea or by air, depending upon circumstances) to the fractionation facilities
- ❒ Cost for serology and NAT testing as required
- ❒ Fractionation charge per unit of product made (e.g. per g of albumin and IgG, and IU of FVIII and FIX), or per litre of plasma fractionated. A minimum guaranteed yield may be associated to the charge
- ❒ Shipment of the products to the country of origin
- ❒ Plasma product registration costs
- ❒ Distribution costs
- ❒ Clinical and marketing/sales expenses
- ❒ Administration and overhead charges

Fig. 3: Prerequisite and economic considerations in approaching contract fractionation as an option. Courtesy of the *Global Collaboration for Blood Safety*.

Table 1: Plasma for fractionation.

Differences between European and U.S. standards		
	European Pharmacopeia	Code of Federal Regulations
Pool serological testing	Mandatory for anti-HIV, anti-HCV, HBsAg	Not mentioned
NAT	Mandatory for HCV on *homogenous pool*	Required for HCV and HIV – focus on *donations*
Procurement method	Recovered from blood and through plasmapheresis	Restricted to plasmapheresis
Freezing	Specifies – 30 °C if used for labile factors, - 20 °C for other products	Specifies – 20°C for all
Storage	- 20 °C – one temperature insult to - 5 °C ≤ 72 h	- 20 °C – one temperature insult to - 5 °C ≤ 72 h, ≥ one temperature insult to + 10 °C requires relabelling
FVIII level	Specified to 0.7 IU/mL	unspecified

point of plasma ignore the irrelevance of this concept to a colloidal solution such as plasma. Studies on the phase transitions undergone by frozen plasma as it warmed indicate the absence of a single eutectic and the presence of a number of transitions accompanied by temperature changes which may have a bearing on the activity of plasma proteins such as coagulation factors [12]. However, while the EP monograph appears to contain a number of requirements, which are scientifically ambiguous, it offers a standard that is applicable to all plasma types irrespective of the procurement method. In the U.S., plasma recovered from whole blood has suffered from an uncertain status, given its lack of recognition on the CFR relative to source plasma. In the European environment, the availability of separate standards for plasma for transfusion and plasma for fractionation addresses some of the issues but the recovery of plasma from whole blood for both purposes leads to some differences (Table 2), which may present difficulties for blood agencies involved in plasma collection. Despite this, such plasma is an important source of plasma for fractionation and continuing processes to rectify its status and integrate it within the regulatory framework internationally are to be strongly encouraged [13].

One such effort ensuing from the voluntary standards proposed by the Plasma Protein Therapeutics Association (PPTA) has recently sharpened the tension between the PPTA and the corresponding organisation in the public-sector-orientated fractionators represented by the European Plasma Fractionation Association (EPFA). The voluntary standards of the PPTA have done much to enhance the safety of plasma raw material from the commercial source plasma sector [14]. However, these standards are orientated to the source plasma industry based upon remunerated donors. In many ways, the environment generating recovered plasma from voluntary whole blood donors is different and some aspects of the PPTA standards are incompatible with this environment. Of note in this aspect is the PPTA's policy of testing a sample of donors for drugs, a policy which, while being difficult to implement in the voluntary whole blood environment, is also scientifically difficult to link to the safety of the final plasma derivatives. Furthermore, studies indicating a high positive rate in such testing in source plasma donors throws doubt on the efficacy of the process [15].

Table 2: European standards for plasma.

Parameter	Council of Europe Guide[1] Plasma for transfusion	European Pharmacopeia[2] Plasma for fractionation
Blood storage	preferably < 6 hours, ≤ 18 hours, if held + 20°C- + 24°C, ≤ 24 hours	for labile protein manufacture, ≤ 24 hours, for non-labile protein manufacture ≤ 72 hours
Plasma freezing	≤ 1 hour, to -30°C	for labile protein manufacture to -30°C within 24 hours of collection, for non-labile protein manufacture -20°C
Screening	all units • anti-HIV1 + 2 • HbsAg • anti-HCV • anti-HBc (if required on WB) • syphilis (if required on WB) • anti-HTLV I + II (if required on WB)	all units • anti-HIV1 + 2 • HBsAg • Anti-HCV Pool testing for HCV RNA & anti-HIV1 + 2, anti-HCV

1 Guide to the preparation, quality assurance and use of blood components 9th edition. Council of Europe publishing 2003.

2 Human plasma for Fractionation. European Pharmacopeia Monograph, European Department for Quality of Medicines 2002.

Overall, the reconciliation of standards for plasma for fractionation remains an urgent issue for regulators and industry alike. The need for a common standard is obvious and urgent. Two meetings of the FDA's Blood Products Advisory Committee (BPAC) addressed the issue and reached the position of proposing to the BPAC a new standard for recovered plasma in the U.S.A. which would have obviated the current (unsatisfactory) situation whereby this product is supplied under the short supply provisions of the CFR. The standards proposed by the FDA and the recovered plasma sector in the U.S.A. are similar in all their crucial points but it is this author's view that both documents fail to address the need for the fractionator to be assured of the raw material's safety to the same extent as is possible through the PPTA's voluntary standards. In this regard, this author is of the opinion that the European concept of the Plasma Master File (PMF) as described by the European Medicines Evaluation Agency (EMEA) provides a good basis for such a standard [16] (Table 3). The essential data are provided independently of the plasma origin, and are such as to allow the regulator to assess the essential safety features, particularly the features contributing to viral safety, independently of issues centred around the need for specific products such as coagulation factors which are considered in the context of standard contracts.

Other aspects of the standards environment contribute significantly to the availability and mobility of plasma. The volume of plasma collected through apheresis is also an issue requiring review and harmonisation. A recent study indicating satisfactory donor health outcomes for donors undergoing plasmapheresis regimens of different intensity should stimulate European authorities to review their currently conservative standards for maximum plasmapheresis volumes [17]. The European Parliament's drive for self-sufficiency through voluntary donation in all blood derivatives drove some members to attempt to exclude products derived from remunerated donors [18], hence any measures which can place current European standards for collection on an evidence base and generate more products should be welcomed by European legislators.

Table 3: Requirements for plasma for fractionation specified in the Plasma Master File.

• Origin of plasma – blood plasma collection establishments – data on epidemiology of infection transmitted by blood: – absence of collection in high prevalence areas
• permanent reassessment of epidemiological data
• selection/exclusion criteria
• screening tests of marker of infection
• system to trace the path of any donation
• Plasma quality – storage and transport – plasma pool preparation – specifications
Standard contracts

Factors Affecting Access to Finished Products

Developments in medical practice and biotechnology

As the clinical practice of transfusion medicine becomes exposed to the tenets of evidence-based medicine, the plasma industry is becoming subject to pressures in maintaining its traditional product portfolio. The effect of the Cochrane review on albumin usage has already been described [1], and has had a severe impact on the product's role as a predominant driver for plasma collection and a major industry earner. Concurrently, the ability to deliver gram amounts of immunoglobulin through intravenous formulations (IVIG) has increased the consumption of this product for the established immunodeficiency indications, and has fuelled an ever-increasing usage for a range of immunomodulatory indications [19], which have contributed to its current role as the driver for plasma procurement in the developed world. While debate on the evidence base for these indications is continuing, it is noteworthy that at least one product delivery process based on an evidence-based review of indications [20] has failed to maintain supply as predicted by the best estimates of plasma requirements and consumption on the basis of approved indications. It is important to note that this occurred in a health care delivery system where IVIG continues to be delivered free of charge, while competitor interventions for the relevant indications are not.

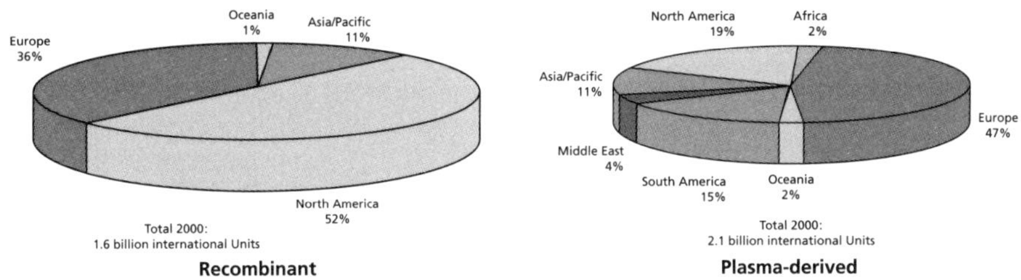

Fig. 4: FVIII distribution 2002. Courtesy: Market Research Bureau 2002.

The predominance of IVIG has been sharpened by the declining use of plasma-derived Factor VIII (FVIII) in the developed markets (Fig. 4). However, the level to which recombinant FVIII rVIII has become established in haemophilia care has not been solely a function of economic factors. The entry of rVIII in Canada, Eire and, to a lesser extent the U.K., has been influenced by health policy decisions which have been retrospectively viewed as faulty by several processes of public inquiry such as the Krever Commission in Canada, the Lindsay Tribunal in Eire and the Phillips Inquiry in the United Kingdom. All these processes occurred in blood systems with a strong commitment to delivering haemophilia care through domestic blood supplies, which led, in many instances, to unfortunate lapses in safety. The issue of self-sufficiency is therefore important in assessing its effect on the viability of the plasma industry.

The "self-sufficiency" movements

The evolution of the concept of self-sufficiency in blood has been reviewed [21]. For the purpose of the current work, it suffices to comment on the effect of the determination of certain health care providers to maintain a capacity to fractionate plasma domestically in circumstances which appear unrelated to standard health care policy tenets. Thus, the U.K. elected to maintain a national fractionation capacity after its decision not to use its own plasma because of a potential risk of variant Creuztfeld Jakob disease (vCJD), to the extent of purchasing a commercial U.S. plasma agency, and maintained its haemophilia population on products derived from this arrangement until its announcement of a full recombinant policy in early 2003. In Japan, self-sufficiency for FVIII has been resolved by the simple expedient of defining it at a level which is not commensurate to the standard of care expected in a first world economy (Fig. 5). While these policies are clearly designed to maintain a domestic capacity to fractionate, their promulgation to the extent of delaying the optimisation of haemophilia care to the level commensurate with the overall socio-economic status of the countries involved is ill-advised. The Krever process [22] led to the near total demise of the Canadian fractionation industry after the revelation that its protection was a significant factor in the unacceptable events described, and prompted Krever to comment:

"The principle of self-sufficiency does not mean that plasma must be fractionated by a domestic fractionation facility."

Therefore, efforts to maintain a fractionation capacity in the face of a good health policy are ill-advised and may obviate the original intention of protecting the domestic industry by hastening its demise in the event of hazardous outcomes.

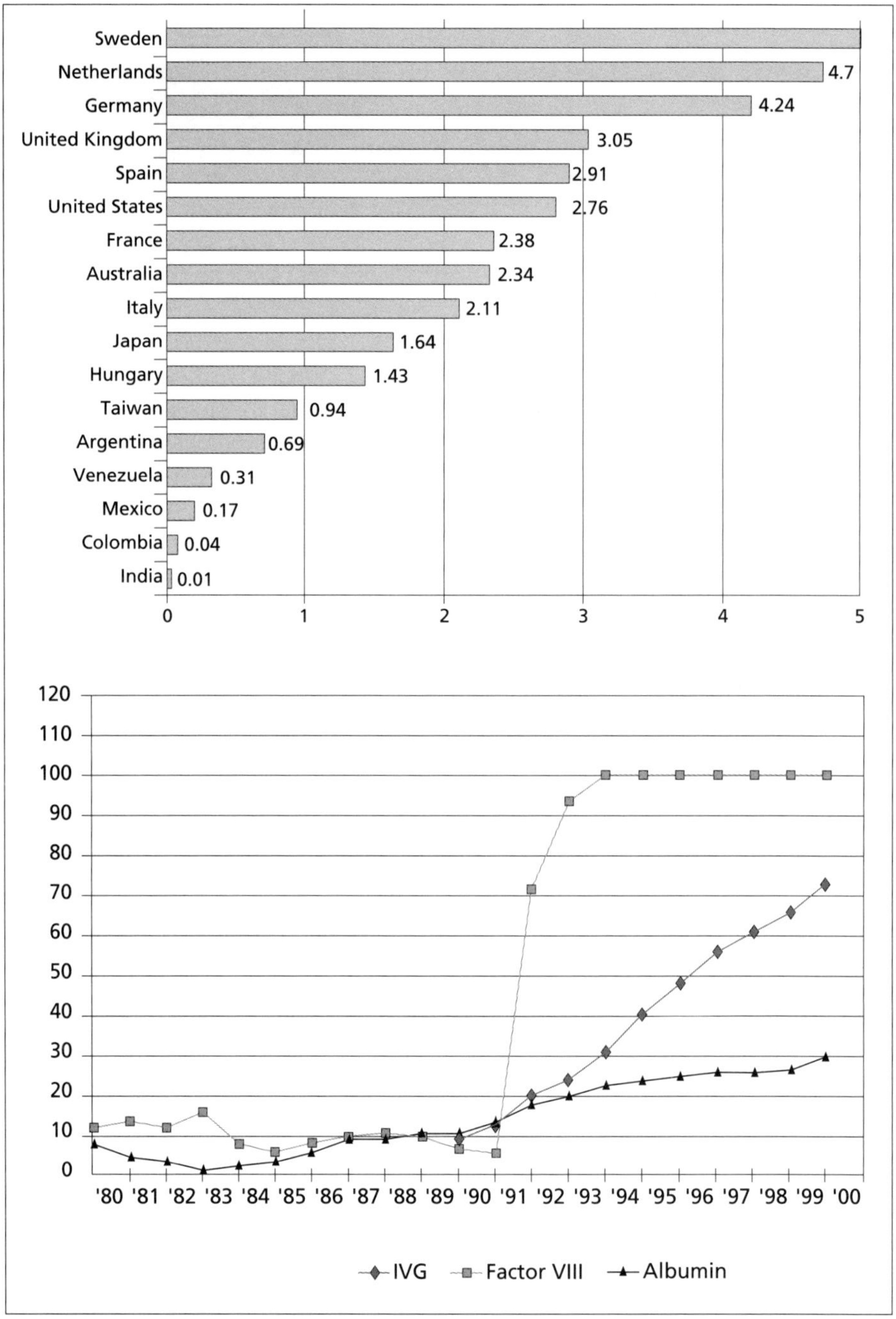

Fig. 5: FVIII supply in Japan. FVIII usage/head of population derived from Market Research Bureau data. Japanese Health Ministry data defines self-sufficiency in FVIII as having been attained in 1998 at a consumption of 1.54 iu/head of population.

Conclusions

While there is a demand for plasma derivatives based on sound evidence and historical experience, the plasma fractionation industry is facing substantial challenges because of technological, clinical and safety factors. Prediction of the industry's demise would be premature and ill-judged, particularly when considering that the majority of the world lacks access to safe and sufficient supplies of important products. Rather than continuing efforts to circumscribe access through nationalistic or economic interests, often cloaked as scientific or ethical principles, the industry, health policy makers and the regulatory framework should increase their efforts to ensure that plasma collection is optimised, that manufacturing principles are improved and that barriers to plasma and product movement are minimised. While plasma continues its sometimes uneasy status as both a gift and a commodity, there is no reason for this to inhibit the industry's future as long as all the players involved realise that the ultimate outcome – health care delivery – is equally addressed through both these features, and maintain their efforts towards that all-important goal.

References

1 Cochrane Injuries Group Albumin Reviewers. Human albumin administration in critically ill patients: systematic review of randomised controlled trials. BMJ 1998; 317: 235-240.

2 Yamey G: Albumin industry launches global propmotion. BMJ 2000; 320: 533.

3 Roberts I, Bunn F: Egg on their faces. The story of human albumin solution. Eval Health Prof 2002; 25: 130-138.

4 Voegler R: The future of plasma protein therapies. Presented at the International Plasma Protein Congress of the Plasma Protein Therapies Association, Brussels March 2003. On http://www.ibc-global.com/MANAGEDEVENTS/pm/PPTA/Conferences/RuediWaeger.pdf.

5 Marketing Research Bureau Inc. The Worldwide Plasma Fractions Market 2002. Orange CT, May 2002.

6 Ibid.

7 de Oliveira G. Brazilian Program of self-sufficiency in blood products – Plasma fractionation abroad. Presented to the 10th International Congress for Drug Regulatory Agencies 2002. Available on http://www.who.int/medicines/library/qsm/icdra02/ppt/Plasma_Fraction.ppt.

8 Statements in Latin American Regulators' Forum organised by the World Federation of Hemophilia organised in Miami USA 2002. Summarised on http://www.wgh.org/content_documents/Newsletters/HW_Dec02_Eng.pdf.

9 Global Collaboration for Blood Safety – World Health Organisation (2003) Information and Fact Sheet – Plasma Contract Fractionation Program. Available on http://www.health.gov.au/bt/index.htm.

10 London Times. Scandal of HIV blood sold as safe by South Africans. 29 August 2000.

11 Joint Committee of Public Accounts and Audit Report no 378 - Chapter 4: Commonwealth management and Regulation of Plasma Fractionation 2001. Available on http://www.aph.gov.au/house/committee/jpaa/agsecond99_00/CHAPTER4.PDF and on http://www.aph.gov.au/hansard/joint/commttee/comjoint.htm.

12 McIntosh RV, Dickson AJ, Smith D, Foster PR: Freezing and thawing plasma, in Cryopreservation and Low Temperature Biology in Blood Transfusion. Dev Haemat Immunol 1990, vol 24, pp 11-24.

13 Callaghan E: Standards for recovered plasma. Presented to the Blood Products Advisory Committee of the FDA June 2002 and June 2003. Available on http://www.fda.gov/OHRMS/DOCKETS/ac/02/briefing/Recovered % 20plasma-BPAC % 206-02.doc and http://www.fda.gov/ohrms/dockets/ac/03/briefing/3961b1_Callaghanrecovered % 20plasma.ppt.

14 Plasma Protein Therapies Association. Voluntary industry standards. On http://www.pptaglobal.org/en/qualitysafety_qseal.cfm.

15 Peters FT, Maurer HH, Hellstern P: Prevalence of illicit drug use in plasmapheresis donors. Vox Sang 2003; 84: 91-95.

16 European Medicines Evaluation Agency. Contribution to part 2.3 of the structure of the dossier for applications for marketing authorisation – Control of starting materials for the production of plasma-derived medicinal products (draft) 2001. On http://www.emea.eu.int/pdfs/human/bwp/205301en.pdf.

17 Helstern P: The safety of long-term serial donor plasmapheresis (SIPLA). Presented at the International Plasma Protein Congress of the Plasma Protein Therapies Association, Brussels March 2003. On http://www.ibcglobal.com/MANAGEDEVENTS/pm/PPTA/Conferences/PeterHelmstern.pdf.

18 Lund T: Sitting of the European Parliament on 5 September 2001 – Quality and safety standards for human blood and blood components. On http://www3.europarl.eu.int/omk/omnsapir.so/debatsL5?FILE=20010905EN & LANGUE = EN & LEVEL = DOC & NUMINT = 3-424.

19 Farrugia A, Poulis P: Intravenous immunoglobulin: regulatroy perspectives on use and supply. Transf Med 2001; 11: 63-74.

20 Report to Australian Health Ministers Advisory Council – Review of use and supply of intravenous immunoglobulin in Australia 2000. On http://www.health.gov.au/hsdd/bodt/pdf/ivig.pdf.

21 The Supply and Safety of Blood and Blood Products - Evidence, risk and policy, in Competing Rationalities: Evidence-Based Health Policy, Oxford University Press, 2003, in press.

22 Report of the Krever Commission of Inquiry into the Blood System in Canada 1996. Available on http://www.hc-sc.gc.ca/english/krever/k_wp_e. html.

Dr. A. Farrugia, Blood & Tissues Unit, Office of Devices, Blood and Tissues, Australian Therapeutic Goods Administration, PO Box 100, Woden, ACT 2606, Australia.
E-mail: Albert.farrugia@health.gov.au

Vyas GN, Williams AE (eds): Advances in Transfusion Safety.
Dev Biol (Basel). Basel, Karger, 2005, vol 120, pp 97-100.

Impact of Source Plasma Standards on Recovered Plasma

C. Bianco

America's Blood Centers, Washington, DC, USA

RECOVERED PLASMA AND SOURCE PLASMA

The core mission of not-for-profit blood centres in the U.S. is to collect whole blood from volunteer donors for distribution to the hospitals and patients they serve. Whole blood is separated into components including red blood cells, platelets and plasma. About 20% of all plasma produced by blood centres is licensed by the U.S. Food and Drug Administration (FDA) as plasma for transfusion into recipients. The remainder is converted into recovered plasma and shipped to fractionators for the manufacture of derivatives (Factor VIII, IX, IVIG, Albumin, Alpha-1 Anti-trypsin, etc.). Each year, about 2.2 million litres of recovered plasma are shipped for further manufacture in the U.S. [1]. Today's recovered plasma fulfils all major FDA criteria required for transfusion into a recipient.

To satisfy the demand for plasma for further manufacture, the FDA has also licensed source plasma, usually obtained by apheresis of paid donors. It is not intended for direct transfusion into recipients and is regulated by the FDA (21 CFR 640.60). About 9.5 million litres of source plasma are collected each year in the U.S. Europe produces about four million litres of recovered plasma and two million litres of source plasma in a year.

Recovered plasma is the only blood component manufactured by FDA-licensed establishments that does not have direct FDA supervision. According to the regulations it is a "by-product derived from Whole Blood collection" and has no expiry date. The collection, preparation, storage and shipping conditions for recovered plasma are dictated by manufacturers of derivatives in a *short supply agreement* signed between each collecting facility and manufacturer. To use the short supply provisions, the licensed derivatives manufacturer must have in place with their supplier ".... such procedures, inspections, tests or other arrangements as well as ensure full compliance with applicable regulations...." (21 CFR 601.22). This concept was created years ago, when plasma was "recovered" from expired whole blood and made into albumin and other products. In the last 10 years, as a result of regulatory actions, collectors improved their quality systems and short supply agreements became far more detailed. More recently, AABB included recovered plasma into their Standards for Blood Banks and blood banking organizations have attempted to work together with the Plasma Protein Therapeutics Association (PPTA), the trade organization of the plasma therapeutics industry, in the development of voluntary standards. In addition, the Council of Europe and the European Community have issued standards and requirements for the collection and preparation of recovered plasma. Thus, despite the absence of direct regulation and licensing by FDA, fractionators incorporate specifications into a "short supply agreement" (age, time to freezing, storage temperature, etc.) and inspect collecting facilities in order to comply with regulatory requirements.

Whole blood collectors dislike the term "recovered plasma" created in the early 1970s because it conveys the impression that it is a less important product. They would prefer names like "plasma", "plasma from whole blood" or "plasma for further manufacture" that identify the component without other implications.

It should be noted that there are some differences between recovered plasma and source plasma in terms of donor screening and deferrals. They are summarized in Table 1. For instance, recovered plasma is tested for antibodies to the core antigen of HBV and is tested by NAT in smaller pools of 1 – 24 samples. Recovered plasma is also subjected to NAT for West Nile Virus. In addition, individuals who have spent five years or more in Continental Europe are deferred from donating whole blood but are acceptable as source plasma donors. This was allowed by FDA after manufacturers demonstrated experimentally that the fractionation process leads to a substantial reduction of spiked prions.

Attempts to Regulate Recovered Plasma

Blood banking organizations in the U.S. have asked that the FDA create a licence for recovered plasma. They have emphasized that recovered plasma is the only

Table 1: Plasma for transfusion and source plasma are subjected to different requirements for screening tests and donor history deferrals.

Test or deferral	Plasma for transfusion	Source plasma	Comments
HBsAg	Yes	Yes	
Antibodies to HIV-1/2	Yes	Yes	
Antibodies to HTLV-I/II	Yes	No	
Antibodies to HCV	Yes	Yes	
Antibodies to HBV core	Yes	No	
NAT for HIV-1	Yes	Yes	Pools 1-24 versus 512->1,000
NAT for HCV	Yes	Yes	Pools 1-24 versus 512->1,000
NAT for HBV	No	Yes	
NAT for West Nile Virus	Yes	No	Under IND, pools 1-16
Syphilis	Yes	Yes*	*Once every four months
Deferral for travel, malaria	Yes	No	
Deferral for travel, vCJD	Yes	Yes for UK**	**Acceptable if lived in Europe

blood component manufactured by FDA-licensed blood establishments that does not have direct FDA supervision. These organizations feel that indirect regulation by short supply agreements is out of pace with the FDA's current application of drug cGMPs to blood establishments. It is also inconsistent with the strict regulation of Source Plasma. Blood centres also made substantial investments in quality systems, software and facilities applied to all blood components, including recovered plasma.

Proposed PPTA Standards for Recovered Plasma

As these activities progressed, PPTA prepared a proposal for standards for recovered plasma modelled after their voluntary standards for source plasma. The proposal generated substantial controversy among blood banking organizations. While the general concepts of Quality Assurance, Traceability, Documented Donor Qualification, and Verifiable Viral Safety proposed by PPTA are similar to those from the FDA and AABB developed for blood components for transfusion into patients, some of the specific requirements are considered incompatible with the manner in which whole blood collecting facilities operate.

To ensure that collecting facilities have a community-based donor population, PPTA requires that donors have a permanent address within 125 miles (200 km) of the collection site (university students and military personnel may provide a temporary local address and proof of their student or military status). The whole blood sector considers this requirement unacceptable because blood is collected from volunteers in organized segments of communities that may be located further away (churches, corporations, universities, other organizations.) In addition, there is concern about the exclusion of commuters in big cities, exclusion of a member of the House of Representatives or Senate that donates at a mobile blood drive in the Capitol, a state governor that donates somewhere else in the state and the relatives of a patient transferred to a tertiary care facility out of the region or out of state.

Another controversial requirement contained in the proposal is the use of PPTA's National Donor Deferral Registry (NDDR). PPTA maintains an NDDR for HIV, HBV, and HCV that must be consulted before accepting an "applicant" donor (a donor who has not donated for a period of six months or more.) Donors testing repeatedly reactive and/or NAT positive for HIV, HCV, and HBV are entered into the NDDR, as are donors admitting to a history of intravenous drug use. PPTA requires a fee per donor for use of the system. FDA-licensed blood centres have more comprehensive deferral files that are integrated with their computer systems and are consulted automatically every time a first time or repeat donor donates and every time a product is released. In the PPTA Internet- based system, donor IDs must be entered manually, one by one, by an operator. There are no computer interfaces. The system does not deal with other deferrals such as syphilis, HTLV-I/II, indefinite deferrals because of travel or medical history, temporary deferrals, etc. After follow-up meetings between the PPTA and blood banking organizations, the requirement for use of the NDDR was removed from the proposed standards.

Collecting organizations continue to negotiate the creation of a Viral Marker Standard with PPTA. The standard would require a regular assessment of the prevalence of infectious disease markers as a measure of performance in the recruitment and maintenance of a low-risk donor base.

The most controversial item in the PPTA proposal, donor screening for drugs of abuse, has been dropped after extensive discussions with the whole blood sector. The proposed standard required opiate testing of an accurate sample of, at the minimum, 7.5% of the units collected and that all donors be informed in advance that their blood may be tested for drugs or opiates. The prevalence of positives among source plasma donors is approximately one in four million. The volunteer donor sector found this requirement unacceptable because of lack of documentation of deterrent value. Actually, the published experience indicates that is has no deterrent value [2].

Impact of Source Plasma Standards on Recovered Plasma

The consequences of application of the same standards to source plasma and recovered plasma are unknown. It is possible that whole blood collectors, unable to comply with the requirements, may stop producing recovered plasma. This may affect the availability of plasma derivatives and increase the cost of other blood components such as red blood cells and platelets. In addition, plasma derivatives distributed in the U.S. and in Europe would be made exclusively from plasma obtained from paid donors

It is to be hoped that all interested parties, whole blood collectors, fractionators and regulatory agencies will come to an agreement on standards for recovered plasma that preserve the safety of recipients and ensure availability of plasma therapies. These standards should not be burdensome. Common sense indicates that plasma fulfilling the requirements for transfusion into recipients is good for fractionation. Licensing of recovered plasma by FDA could be simplified if the Agency allowed the conversion of plasma for transfusion separated from whole blood or collected by apheresis into licensed plasma for further manufacture. This was actually recommended by the FDA Blood Products Advisory Committee. Short supply agreements would be replaced by contracts defining special requirements for collection, storage and transportation (e.g. time to freeze, storage temperature, etc.) based on fractionators' specifications.

The FDA could also provide a mechanism to allow the shipment for further manufacture of certain plasmas that do not qualify for transfusion in order to meet manufacturers' requirements and increase plasma availability. For instance, plasma derived from whole blood that is reactive for antibodies to the core antigen of hepatitis B is needed to guarantee minimum levels of antibodies to ensure final product safety. Also, plasma from individuals who travelled to a malarial area can safely be used for further manufacture because the parasite does not survive fractionation. To protect blood donors, the new regulation allowing shipment of plasma for transfusion for further manufacture would only apply to infrequent whole blood and plasma collections currently licensed by FDA. FDA would continue to require source plasma licences for establishments that perform frequent plasmapheresis.

References

1 International Blood and Plasma News. The Marketing Research Bureau, Inc. page 128, April 2003.

2 Yamaguchi R, Johnston LD, O'Malley PM: Relationship between student illicit drug use and school drug-testing policies. J Sch Health 2003;73(4):159-164.

Dr. C. Bianco, America's Blood Centers, 725 15th Street, Washington, DC 2005, U.S.A.
E-mail: cbianco@americasblood.org

Vyas GN, Williams AE (eds): Advances in Transfusion Safety.
Dev Biol (Basel). Basel, Karger, 2005, vol 120, pp 101-111.

Perspectives of Paid Whole and Plasma Donation

V. Kretschmer, M. Weippert-Kretschmer, J. Slonka, R. Karger, T. Zeiler

Institute of Transfusion Medicine and Haemostaseology, University Hospital Marburg, Germany

Key words: Voluntary, non-remunerated blood donor; paid donor; transfusion risk; blood supply.

Abstract: Although payment of blood donors is rejected by the WHO, the FDA, the EU, and the Red Cross (RC), in Germany, monetary compensation of expenses is permitted not only for plasmapheresis but also for whole blood donation. The structure and organisation of the institutions ensuring the blood supply in Germany and the pertaining aspects of blood safety will be discussed. Data reported to the health authorities show that the frequency of transfusion-transmitted infection markers in the German donor population is low and that only very few infections have been transmitted through blood. This is underlined by a detailed analysis of the paid donor population of a small university blood service (UBS). The analysis documents a very stable and reliable cohort of predominantly repeat donors. Unpaid RC donors of blood units transfused to patients at the university hospital of Marburg showed a sixteen-times higher sero-conversion rate than those of the UBS ($p < 0.0001$). However, in a survey, 77% of the paid donors denied continuation of blood donation in the event of payment being stopped. Therefore non-remuneration would result in acute blood supply shortages. Since increased blood shortages are to be expected anyway in the near future, all measures improving the supply of safe blood, including monetary compensation, should be objectively discussed without prejudice.

INTRODUCTION

Many reports with more or less valid data have been published, proclaiming that blood and blood components of paid donors bear a higher risk of transfusion-transmissible infections (TTI) than those of unpaid donors [1,2]. The sense of responsibility of donors towards the safety of donated blood may decrease with the growing perception of blood donation as a means to earn money, therefore possibly leading to the denial of any reasons disqualifying blood donation. In addition, following Titmuss's publication in 1970, the altruistic motivation of giving blood of voluntary and non-remunerated donors was proclaimed as a means of maintaining a sense of community in an increasingly individualised society [3]. Consistently, WHO, FDA, EC, EU and particularly the Red Cross banished paid blood donation in their guidelines, directives and statements. Thus, under these circumstances, advocating paid blood donation seems to be inappropriate, at least. Nevertheless, monetary compensation of expenses with a fixed amount of money is common among community and university blood services in Germany. The amount given has remained almost unchanged for the last 40 years although its purchasing power has decreased to about one fifth. Payment of a monetary compensation of 25 Euro for whole blood donation has been allowed by law since 1998 in Germany [4]. Although this compensation is not regarded as payment in a strict sense, it clearly has to be if the definition of the FDA is applied [5]. Therefore, the term "paid donors" is used for remunerated German donors throughout this article.

The growing general concern about increasing blood supply shortages requires an objective discussion of all measures without prejudice aimed at providing the demand for safe blood and blood components [6,7]. Therefore, even payment of donors has to be reconsidered. This article will demonstrate that payment of blood donors does not inevitably result in an increased risk of TTI, at least in Germany, and when tailored donor recruitment procedures are applied.

Organisation of the Blood Supply in Germany

Three different donation systems exist in Germany:

1. Red Cross Blood Services (RCBS)

The RCBS are independent organisations under the umbrella of the German Red Cross (RC). After several mergers, there are currently still six RCBS with in total 35 institutes providing about 70 % of the blood supply (approx. three million whole blood donations per year). Most RCBS are not affiliated to hospitals, and collect blood all over the country, mainly with mobile teams, and are thereby heavily supported by voluntary workers of the respective local RC. A very important aspect with regard to the safety of the donations is that most of the blood is drawn from the rural population. Whole blood donors are mostly, but not always (e.g. in Berlin !), unpaid. In contrast, apheresis donors usually receive a monetary compensation. RCBS produce blood components and plasma products which are sold to hospitals all over the country. The price is set by the RCBS themselves and differs considerably between the various organisations. There is a strong tendency to centralization and takeovers of hospital-based blood services, and there is even a competition for donors and market share between the Red Cross and other blood services.

2. University and Community Blood Services (UCBS)

There is a steadily decreasing number of UCBS (75 in 2002) providing about 30 % of the national blood supply. The UCBS are always departments of hospitals, draw blood mainly at fixed sites in the cities, particularly in the big cities, and almost always pay their donors. The blood components are primarily produced for the hospitals the UCBS are affiliated to. They carry out a higher proportion of platelet- and plasmapheresis, as well as autologous blood donations than the RCBS. Currently, they are becoming increasingly involved in stem-cell separation and storage. All immunohaematological diagnostics in connection with blood transfusion is performed in the laboratories of the UCBS. In addition, a major responsibility of the UCBS consists of consulting clinicians in haemotherapy, and maintaining quality assurance and management in the respective hospitals.

3. Commercial Plasmapheresis Centres (CPC)

Forty-four industrial or private CPC produce about 65 % of source plasma (in 2002: 1.1 million litres) necessary for the industrial production of plasma derivatives. The CPC are usually located in the cities, and draw plasma from paid donors at fixed sites. Because the German rules [8] allow the collection of up to 25 litres per donor per year, frequent donations are possible. A few CPC also sell plasma for direct therapeutic purposes and in addition perform a small number of whole blood donations. Donors are often recruited by advertisements openly offering payment.

Safety of the Blood Supply in Germany

Table 1 shows the prevalence and sero-conversion rate of TTI markers in first-time and repeat whole blood (WB) and plasma (PP) donors as reported to the Robert-Koch-Institut (RKI), the senior federal authority for national infectious disease monitoring (Dr. Ruth Offergeld, Robert-Koch Institute, personal communication 2003). The data clearly show the well-known fact of a significantly higher prevalence of TTI markers in first-time donors than the sero-conversion rate in repeat donors. Compared to other industrialised countries, the rate of positive TTI markers in German donors is rather low. The data for the plasma donors do not seem to be very different from those of the whole blood donors. However, since the rates are related to the number of donations, they have to be multiplied by 10 to 20 if the incidence of TTI markers in this donor population is to be determined. Thus, donors of commercial plasmapheresis centres unquestionably have a clearly higher rate of TTI markers. However, with regard to the infectious load of a given plasma pool used as a source for fractionation, there is no great difference in plasma of WB donation, particularly when the three-times higher volume per plasma donation is taken into account.

Table 1: Infection rates in whole blood (WB) and plasmapheresis (PP) donations (per 100,000) in 2001 reported to Robert Koch Institute (RKI) [R. Offergeld, RKI, personal communication 2003).

Infections	Proven by	First-time donors WB/PP	Repeat donors WB/PP
HIV	EIA + and Westernblot + and/or NAT +	4.7 / 12.7	0.5/0.6
HCV	EIA + and Immunoblot + and/or NAT +	94.5/98.7	1.6/0.7
HBV	HBsAg + and supplement test + and/or NAT +	158.9/73.2	1.4/0.6

In Germany, all suspected TTI and the results of previous investigations have to be reported to the Paul-Ehrlich-Institute, the senior regulatory authority responsible for the procurement and safety of blood and blood products. Figure 1 shows that the number of TTI has never been high in Germany compared to other industrialised countries and has even been reduced substantially during the last few years (Dr. Brigitte Keller-Stanislawski, Paul-Ehrlich Institute, personal communication 2003). Since HIV testing of donors was introduced in 1985 only 11 HIV infections (five since 1995) have been reported, probably due to transfusions. Besides one case in 1986 (blood unit delivered by mistake) and one case in 1992 (test failure), all infections occurred during the window period. After introduction of the HCV-ELISA in 1991 a total of 43 probable HCV TTI have been reported to the PEI. After the introduction of obligatory HCV-NAT testing in Germany in 1998, no more HCV TTI have been reported so far. Eight out of 11 cases in 1998 were attributed to the donations of one plasmapheresis donor of a private plasmapheresis unit who had offended against medical standards.

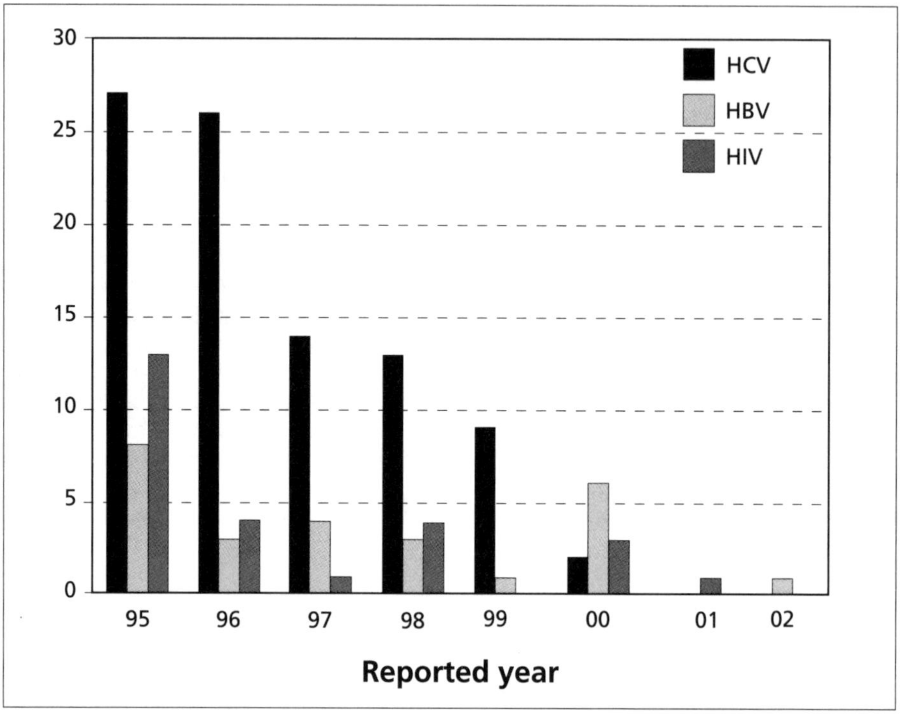

Fig. 1: Transfusion transmittable infections reported to Paul-Ehrlich Institute (PEI) since 1995 with transfusion as probable cause [B. Keller-Stanislawski, PEI, personal communication 2003].

Data of the University Blood Service (UBS) Marburg

Donor population

Marburg is a small town located in the centre of Germany with about 75,000 residents, 20,000 of whom are university students. The UBS carries out about 12,000 whole blood donations, 1,000 plateletphereses, and 5,000 plasmaphereses per year. Approximately 10,000 additional red cell concentrates have to be bought from the RCBS Hessen every year. The UBS performs the complete infectious disease and immunohaematological testing for the blood service, and the complete haemostaseological and immunohaematological diagnostics for the university hospital. Like the other UBSC, the UBS Marburg does not offer money in donor recruitment campaigns. Individuals willing to give blood, the so-called "would-be" donors, are only examined, do not give blood or get money at their first appearance. Half of the donors (Table 2) are university students, most of whom leave Marburg after having finished university. The percentage of unemployed donors is remarkably low when compared with the general unemployment rate in this area at the time when this analysis was carried out. Women make up more than 55.2 % of the "would-be" donors, but have a higher deferral rate mainly due to low haemoglobin values. Therefore, only one third of the actual donors are women. 10.2 % of the donors donate only once, 12.4 % between two to four times, and 77.4 % more than four times. Table 3 shows the "drop-out" rate (deferral and/or non-reappearance) of all "would-be" donors between 1997 and 2000. 9.7 % of the whole blood donations stem from first-time donors (donating their first blood unit when coming the second time). 28.2 % of the WB donations come from donors who have already given blood two to five times, and 26.3 % from donors having donated already 6-10 times. 45.8 % of WB donations stem from donors having donated WB more than 10 times already. The average donation frequency per year is 2.7 WB units (males 3 units, females 2.3 units). It can be concluded from these data that the donor population of the UBS Marburg is very stable and reliable, and that the blood supply is mainly provided by repeat donors who are generally considered to have a clearly lower rate of TTI markers than first-time donors, the more so as this rate is expected to decrease further with the number of donations increasing.

Table 2: Social status of donors in Marburg.

Students	52.7 %
University graduates	7.7 %
Office worker/officials	17.3 %
Workmen	6.9 %
Workers	5.8 %
Housewives	3.8 %
Others	3.1 %
Unemployed	2.9 %*

* Official rate of unemployed in this area ca. 8.2 %.

Table 3: Drop-out rate of donors starting between 1997 and 2000 (whole blood donations until 2003).

Donor status	**Number**	**Loss [%]**
Would be donors	4,924	
Accepted as donors	4,385	10.9
Coming to 1st donation	3,407	25.9
Released 1st donations	3,250	4.6
Mean loss per donation		15.6 ± 3.9
Mean loss by selection		4.5 ± 1.8

Survey on monetary compensation

In 1994, an intense debate about whether it was advisable and feasible to abandon payment of blood donors was going on. This prompted us to perform a survey on our donors' attitudes towards monetary compensation [9]. During a two-month period a questionnaire was handed to our WB donors that took no more than five minutes to be answered. A confidential and anonymous atmosphere was guaranteed. 1157 (95.2 %) of 1215 questionnaires were returned and analysed. 21.4 % or 31.1 % of the donors did not agree to money transfer to a bank account or accepted non-negotiable cheques, respectively. The same percentage indicated they would stop further donation if these measures were implemented (21.7 % and 30.5 %, respectively). Monetary compensation with tickets or coupons for cinema, concerts, theatre or restaurants was not accepted by 72.7 %, and at least 61.1 % stated they would not continue giving blood. 86.1 % did not agree to general cancellation of money compensation, and only 23 % indicated they would continue to donate blood. Refusal of non-payment was quite comparable between different professions and level of education (Table 4). Surprisingly, soldiers and the unemployed, as well as university graduates and students, showed the highest willingness to continue blood donation without any monetary compensation. Even though the percentage of these donors was low and amounted to only one third in these respective groups, it was remarkably higher than the 12 % of housewives who stated they would continue giving blood without any monetary compensation. It was also surprising that the refusal of non-payment increased with age, e.g. 75.8 % in donors 18 to 21 years old against 87.1 % in donors 41 to 65 years old, and the number of previous donations (first-time donors 70.7 %, > 4 donations 78.5 %).

Although it cannot simply be concluded from this survey that 77 % of paid donors would discontinue giving blood if monetary compensation were withdrawn, it is realistic to expect a loss of at least 50 % and a considerable reduction in the donation frequency of the remaining donors. Therefore, cancellation of payment would result in acute shortages in the blood supply. Money is obviously taken for granted by our donors, and this attitude seems especially to be linked to the willingness to be a loyal repeat donor.

Table 4: Marburg survey: refusal of nonpayment and discontinuation of donation in case of cancellation of payment [9].

Social status	Denial [%]	Discontinuation [%]
Students	86.6	71.8
University graduates	85.7	68.6
Office worker/officials	86.8	82.1
Workmen	93.1	90.3
Workers	83.3	80.8
Housewives	93.3	88.2
Soldiers	100	68.6
Unemployed	100	66.7

Safety of the blood supply in Marburg

The question whether these donors provide safe blood can only be answered on the basis of the frequency of donor sero-conversions and positive look-back investigations in case of infected recipients of blood. Because one third of the blood units used in our hospital stems from the RCBS, a direct comparison between the donors of the RCBS and our donors is possible (Table 5). Since 1994, in the UBS Marburg, 17 look-back procedures had to be performed because of sero-conversion of donors of blood that had been administered to patients in our hospital; in 15 cases donors of the RCBS, in two cases donor of the UBS Marburg were involved. In relation to the total number of blood units administered, the sero-conversion rate in the RCBS donors was about 16 times higher. The difference was highly significant ($p < 0.0001$, χ^2-test). Even when a two to three times higher donation rate of the USB donors is taken into account a significant difference in favour of the USB donors in Marburg remains. This is consistent with the results of the look-back procedures that had to be initiated because recipients had sero-converted. In eight out of 10 cases blood transfusion could be excluded as the cause of the infection. In two cases the donors also had sero-converted meanwhile, both of them from the RCBS. In summary, the blood of the paid donors of our institution is at least as safe as that from unpaid donors of the RCBS.

Table 5: Look back procedures since 1994 because of sero-converted donors of blood units administered to patients of the university hospital Marburg (*χ^2).

	RCBS	Marburg	p-value*
Blood units	**86,331**	**179,426**	
Sero-converted donors			
Total	15	2	< 0.0001
HIV	3	1	n.t.
HBV	3	0	n.t.
HCV	9	1	n.t.

n.t. = not tested

Discussion

Since around 1960 there has been increasing concern about payment of blood donors owing to a large number of reports proclaiming that blood and blood components of paid donors bear a higher risk of TTI than those of unpaid donors. However, most of the published data are not suited to demonstrate conclusively that payment of WB donors inevitably increases this risk. In 1998, Eastlund presented an overview of the majority of publications on this topic [1]. He admitted that many of these studies involved only a small number of subjects, were neither prospective nor well controlled, and lacked statistical testing. However, he concluded that the preponderance of the reported data showed that monetary inducement of blood donation is associated with a higher prevalence of TTI in donors, an increased number of contaminated blood components, and an increased transmission of viral infections to recipients. He still conceded that the accuracy and generalization of these conclusions may have been limited because of the methodological flaws of many of the studies quoted. He also mentioned that a higher prevalence of TTI in paid donors was not a universal finding. Therefore, he put particular emphasis on other benefits of an all-volunteer system "which may foster social ties and community solidarity".

Van der Poel and co-workers recently presented an update of the published data and calculated the relative risk of TTI from paid versus unpaid donors [2]. They included 28 data sets in their analysis and found a significantly higher risk of TTI in paid donors. Like Eastlund, they compared paid PP donors with non-paid WB donors which is completely unacceptable with regard to the determination of the risk of TTI originating from paid WB donation. PP donors mostly undergo frequent plasma donation. There is no doubt that advertising for plasma donation by offering money regularly up to once or twice a week may attract the wrong population and, in addition, may cause some economic dependence which prevents self-exclusion on health grounds. The data from the RKI referred to above show that the frequency of TTI markers is clearly higher in plasma donors. The analysis of van der Poel et al. still includes reports based on unconfirmed test results and invalid statistics. Although various studies were based on different concepts, and were only rarely controlled for confounding factors such as geographical differences and other population characteristics (e. g. age, gender and social status), the authors argue that bias had not systematically influenced the overall assessment [10]. Even a publication bias has to be considered. Because payment of blood donors is banned in the leading parts of the world it can be assumed that data in accordance with accepted conventional opinion might be easier to publish. Offergeld and Burger from the RKI state that the analysis of van der Poel and colleagues offended against current standards of epidemiological research [10].

In the analysis of van der Poel et al the recently published data of only HCV-NAT-positive donors in Germany is of particular importance because these data should be suited to represent the TTI risk of paid and unpaid donors during the window period. The authors calculated from these data an 8.4 times higher relative risk for TTI originating from paid UCBS donors in comparison to unpaid RCBS donors in Germany. However, the authors did not discuss the background of these data. Hitzler presented the UCBS data at the IABs meeting in Frankfurt in 2001 to demonstrate that general HCV-NAT testing might be helpful to detect infected donors during the window period, but the data had not been gathered to describe the current epidemiological situation of HCV in UCBS donors [11]. The UCBS have resisted general HCV-NAT testing for a long time because of its questionable cost-effectiveness [12]. Therefore, most of the UCBS started with HCV-NAT testing only shortly before it became obligatory in 1998, whereas the RCBS had already routinely applied HCV-NAT testing for several years. Therefore, the HCV-NAT data of the UCBS were not fully reliable, a problem the Red Cross of North Rhine-Westphalia had also faced a couple of years ago. A number of only HCV-NAT positive donors never sero-converted. In addition, the data were incomplete because only 43 % of the UCBS reported their figures. The data mainly came from blood services in cities with a high prevalence of TTI markers which felt a greater pressure to start HCV-NAT testing as soon as possible.

Apart from these and other drawbacks, reservations about the conclusions of van der Poel and colleagues are predominantly warranted because the authors did not take into account the extreme geographic differences in the distribution of

RCBS and UCBS and their respective donors. For example, the considerable geographic differences in the distribution of HIV in Germany reflect this situation for TTI. The frequency of AIDS differs four- to 40-fold between the regions in the East of Germany and the big cities such as Western Berlin, Hamburg, Düsseldorf, Cologne, Frankfurt or Munich [13]. After the German unification, the RCBS have taken over nearly all blood services in the East. In addition, the RCBS draw blood primarily from the rural population, whereas the UCBS draw blood primarily in the cities. Although the discussion has focused on HCV, the distribution of AIDS is even more relevant for assessing the TTI risk emanating from paid WB donors because the reservation about payment for blood donation are especially directed against a sub-group of the population with an increased risk of all TTI. The distribution of HCV in Germany, even though not based on comparably valid data, also shows considerable differences between the various federal states. Again, the states in the East of Germany, on average, have a clearly lower frequency of hepatitis C than most of the other states in Germany [14]. Therefore, the conclusions drawn by van der Poel et al. concerning payment of donors in Germany lack a valid foundation.

In contrast, our data show that paid donors at our institution are at least as safe as unpaid donors of the RCBS. Furthermore, it can be concluded that payment of donors can generally be made as safe as unpaid donation in an economically and socially well-balanced system. This has already been shown by others when preselected apheresis donors and unpaid WB donors were compared [15,16]. However, payment of WB donors requires taking appropriate precautions:

- There should be no advertising by offering money, in order to prevent recruitment of donors in urgent need of money. The amount given must not be too high in relation to income support and cost of living. In a socially well-balanced society remuneration is only regarded as a compensation for travel expenses etc. as many voluntary workers also obtain and expect.
- Upon their first appearance at the blood centre, people willing to donate blood should only undergo a medical examination; no blood donation and no monetary compensation should take place. This excludes individuals who need money immediately, e.g. drug addicts. In addition, people who only want to have an HIV test will also not return, a problem faced by institutions only recruiting unpaid donors as well.
- The examination should be carried out thoroughly and confidentially by well-educated and trained medical staff who make their decision whether or not to accept a certain donor as responsibly as possible.
- The donors have to be thoroughly informed about the risks they represent for the recipients if they do not collaborate responsibly in the health examination process.
- The donors should be invited to donation by post. This excludes donors with no fixed abode. Occasional large-scale donation events do not allow the conditions outlined above to be fulfilled, and also preclude a familiarization process which is the best way to motivate donors to repeat donation.
- Moreover, confidential unit-exclusion not leading to the denial of the monetary compensation also contributes to the safety of paid blood donation. Furthermore,

repeat donors who have not given blood for a year or more should be dealt with as if they were new donors, performing only an examination on their first appearance.

- Finally, we firmly advocate a central donor deferral system which cannot be enforced in Germany, though, because of special national rights of privacy protection.

At least in Germany it appears to be totally impossible to collect enough source plasma by plasmapheresis without payment. Thus, even the RCBS pay plasmapheresis donors. To prevent recruitment of high(er)-risk donors plasmapheresis units should be integrated into RCBS or UCBS and should carry out plasmithereses in a mixed donation programme. i.e. donors should be enrolled only after having proved their reliability as WB donors and should undergo plasmaphereses only for limited time intervals followed by WB donations. Fixed appointments not only facilitate organization of the plasmapheresis unit, they may also help to assess the reliability of the donors better. The programme of the American Blood Resources Association (ABRA) with its supplementation goes in the right direction [6].

What are the general perspectives of paid blood donation? We are living in an increasingly economically oriented world. Most voluntary workers, at least in Western Europe, get monetary compensation, which does not mean that they have no altruistic motivation. Blood donation in itself, i.e. without any monetary compensation, is undoubtedly rather attractive in small communities where everybody knows each other, where the priest, the schoolteacher, the mayor or the neighbours see one donating blood, especially when giving for the 10th time and being honoured with a pin. However, in contrast to the rural population, city dwellers have neither enough sense of community nor are they interested in honorary rewards in order to give blood at all. Therefore, payment may appeal to an additional donor population and may help to retain repeat donors. On the other hand, every kind of incentive, regardless of its economic value, can become inappropriately attractive, e.g. if especially idolized. The fact that this attraction may be variable among individuals makes different incentives even more difficult to compare with regard to their risk of attracting high(er)-risk donors. Furthermore, blood banking and blood component production have become a business in which many people and institutions earn a great deal of money. Why do we expect that the donor is the only altruistic link in this economic chain? Therefore, somewhat provocatively, how can a constant blood supply be ensured with only unpaid donors when the public is being told by the media that the blood supply is a huge business?

Whenever there were scandals relating to blood banking in Germany, e.g. because blood was sold to the U.S. even in times of blood shortage or unconscionable salaries of blood bank directors were reported, the willingness to donate at the blood services concerned dramatically decreased, and the blood supply was at risk. On the other hand, as our own experience shows, the risks attributed to the payment of blood donors can be estimated and be largely avoided. In conclusion, we think a dual system with paid and unpaid donors is more effective and can be made as safe as a system with only unpaid donors. However, we need more scientific evidence about the motivation of the various people in different countries and regions, with different cultures, religion, economic and social circumstances, etc. We cannot transfer our results and conclusions anywhere else. Conversely, other nations should not transfer their experience or even only belief to the situation in Germany.

References

1 Eastlund T: Monetary blood donation incentives and the risk of transfusion-transmitted infection. Transfusion 1998; 38: 874-882.

2 Poel van der CL, Seifried E, Schaasberg WP: Paying for blood donations: still a risk? Vox Sang 2002; 83: 285-293.

3 Titmuss R: The gift relationship: from human blood to social policy. Allen and Unwin, London 1970.

4 Gesetz zur Regelung des Transfusionswesens (TFG) vom 1. Juli 1998 (BGBl. I, S. 1752) Gesetzestext und Begründung der Bundesregierung vom 13.01.1998. BT Drcks. 13/9594.

5 U.S. Food and Drug Administration. CPG Sec. 230.150 Blood donor classification statement: paid or voluntary donor. 2002; http:/www.fda.gov/ora/compliance_ref/cpg/cpgbio/cpg230-150final. htmtion

6 Simon TL. Monetary compensation for plasma donors: a record of safety, Transfusion 1998; 38: 883-886.

7 Simon TL: Where have all the donors gone? A personal reflection on the crisis in America's volunteer blood program. Transfusion 2003; 43: 273-279.

8 Wissenschaftlicher Beirat der Bundesärztekammer und Paul-Ehrlich Institut: Richtlinien zur Gewinnung von Blut und Blutbestandteilen und zur Anwendung von Blutprodukten (Hämotherapie). Bundesgesundheitsblatt 2000; 43 (7): 555-589.

9 Zeiler T, Kretschmer V: Blutspenderbefragung zum Thema "Aufwandsentschädigung für Blutspender". Infusionsther Transfusionsmed 1995; 22:19-24.

10 Offergeld R, Burger R. Remuneration of blood donors and its impact on transfusion safety. Vox Sang 2003; 85: 49 (Letter).

11 Seifried E, Hitzler W: Status of NAT screening for HCV, HIV and HBV: experience in Germany. Infus Ther Transfus Med 2001; 28: 231 (Abstract).

12 Kretschmer V, Sibrowski W, Bein G, Gürtler L: Testung auf HIV-1-, HBV- und HCV-Genome mit Nukleinsäure-Amplifikationstechniken bei Erythrozytenkonzentraten. Infusionsther Transfusionsmed 1997; 24: 125-129.

13 Robert Koch Institut. Epidemiologisches Bulletin 2003/Sonderausgabe A, p 9.

14 Robert Koch Institut. Infektionsepidemiologisches Jahrbuch meldepflichtiger Krankheiten für 2001. Mercedes-Druck, Berlin 2002, pp 69-71.

15 Taswell HF: Directed, paid and self-donors; in Clark GM (ed): Competition in Blood Services, Arlington, American Association of Blood Banks, 1987, pp 137-148.

16 Strauss RG, Ludwig GA, Smith PJ, et al: Concurrent comparison of the safety of paid cytopheresis and volunteer whole blood donors. Transfusion 1994; 34: 116-121.

Dr. V. Kretschmer, Institute of Transfusion Medicine and Haemostaseology, University Hospital, Conradistrasse, D-35033 Marburg, Germany.
E-mail: kretschv@mailer.uni-marburg.de

Vyas GN, Williams AE (eds): Advances in Transfusion Safety.
Dev Biol (Basel). Basel, Karger, 2005, vol 120, pp 113-117.

Perspectives on Compensated Plasma Donation

J.M. Bult

Plasma Protein Therapeutics Association (PPTA), Annapolis, MD, USA

Abstract: The subject of compensating donors has been and sometimes still is a topic for lively discussion. It is my view that compensating plasma donors for their time and effort is appropriate when done in a well regulated environment. I will attempt in this presentation to outline the reasons why this is the case.

INTRODUCTION

Over a million of people in the world often depend on lifesaving therapies made from human blood or plasma, whether these are transfusions with (red) blood components or therapies made from human plasma. However, there are distinct differences between blood and plasma therapies due to contrasting collection, preparation/manufacturing, safety and distribution practices.

Whole blood can be collected several times per year from a donor (from males more frequently then from females). The frequency of donation varies depending on national regulations, but several reports put the average donation per donor at once or twice per year. The average collected volume of whole blood is about 250 ml in a procedure that takes up to 30 minutes. Most whole blood donations are used for transfusion purposes in a hospital setting. In cases when the collected whole blood is not used for direct transfusion, it can be made available for the manufacture of finished products. Plasma collected in this manner is called recovered plasma.

Plasma can be donated more frequently. The plasma donation is done through an automated procedure called plasmapheresis. The procedure normally takes one and a half to two hours. During this procedure, the red cells are separated from the plasma and returned to the donor immediately. The frequency of donation can be higher because plasma regeneration takes place within 24 hours. The average frequency for a plasma donor in the U.S.A. is 17 times per year [1]. The frequency is restricted by national regulations. In the United States a donor can donate up to twice a week, whereas in Europe donation is restricted to once per week or every other week with maximum volumes between 15 and 25 litres per year. The volumes per donation vary between 450 ml and 830 ml.

Compensation

The average compensation for the time and efforts related to a regular plasma donation in the United States is $15 to $20. In Germany a compensation up to 25 Euro is given and acceptable by law for both plasma and blood donations. However, many blood donors receive other forms of compensation, such as reimbursement of travel costs, time off work and other tokens of appreciation. Time off work can take two full days. In addition, there are many examples in different countries where blood donors receive T-shirts, tickets for events, discounts on medical services, free Internet use, telephone cards and so on.

In my view these are acceptable practices because it is justified to recognize donors for their willingness to help someone else. It seems strange to me that some people believe that a financial compensation is unacceptable, whereas the forms of compensation described above can easily exceed the averages that are acceptable in our industry. For me, both forms are appropriate and should be encouraged. We are transparent in what we do and believe and are proud that we have so many volunteer compensated donors. In 2002, the approximately 450 collection centres associated with PPTA collected over 13 million litres of plasma.

In the United States, Germany, Austria and Sweden, plasma donors can be compensated for their time and efforts related to the donation. It is no wonder that these countries have the most successful plasma collection programmes in the world and contribute considerably when it comes to the availability of plasma that is so needed for the manufacture of life-saving plasma-derived therapies.

Voluntary or Not?

Each donation is done out of free will and is in my perception therefore a voluntary donation. No individual is forced to donate. Sometimes the suggestion is made that a blood donation is voluntary and a plasma donation is not. This shows disrespect for the plasma donors, many of whom may have the same altruistic reasons to donate that blood donors have. The term "voluntary compensated donor" is a factual description of the reality of the donors we work with. Some have expressed criticism for using that term because it was felt that the use of the word voluntary should only be used for blood donors. It is obvious that I do not share this approach.

Differences in Donor Screening

Before donating, each blood donor receives a physical examination that includes blood pressure and haemoglobin tests. Each blood donation is then checked for different pathogen markers, including HIV, HBV and HCV. This procedure is repeated at every donation. Individuals who donate more than once are called repeat donors by the whole blood community, independent from the interdonation interval. Even when this interval is five years or more, the blood donor is still considered to be a repeat donor.

The procedure to become a plasma donor is quite different. When an individual attempts to donate plasma in the United States their name is first checked against the National Donor Deferral Registry (NDDR) to ascertain whether that individual has been deferred from donating in the past for a positive viral screening for HIV, HBV or HCV. If that is the case, then the person cannot be accepted as a donor.

Once a potential plasma donor has been cleared through the NDDR they are given a full medical examination and tested for viral markers. If the results from that test are negative, meaning that no signs of viral infection can be detected, then the individual (then called applicant donor) has to come back to undergo the whole procedure again at a different time. Only a person who successfully passes the screening twice at different times becomes a Qualified Donor. When a donor does not return within six months for another donation, the procedure starts all over again.

The Qualified Donor standard effectively eliminates these so-called "test-seekers". These individuals are only interested in test-results and use the donation process as an easy way to obtain these results. As one can imagine, we are not interested in these individuals becoming donors.

Truthful Information?

Sometimes it is suggested that the promise of monetary compensation can increase the risk that donors will lie or withhold information during the initial screen process. Dr. Simon wrote about this subject recently in an article. I quote: "The concept that paid donors are a less safe source of blood for transfusion than volunteer donors is based on very old data. Often the assumption that people would be untruthful in answering the blood donor questionnaire to receive payment is cited. There is no evidence that this occurs with any greater frequency than untruthfulness due to social pressure among volunteers." [2].

Ethics

Is it ethical to compensate plasma donors monetarily? This is often determined by cultural and educational differences. The French ethical philosophy may differ from the Anglo-Saxon philosophy, which in turn can be different from the Japanese philosophy. Our members believe that it is absolutely ethically acceptable that an individual be compensated for their time and effort for a plasma donation procedure, as long as it is done in a strict regulated environment set by competent regulatory authorities. Compensation for a donation without the existence of a strict regulatory environment to cover blood- and/or plasma donations should not be encouraged.

The underlying ethical principle that everybody agrees with is to do no harm. Doing no harm also means that therapies should be made available for patients all over the world who are in need of these sometimes live-saving therapies. From that perspective there is no difference whether therapies are made from compensated donations or not. Compensation of a donor does not harm the donor or the patient. The European Medicines Evaluation Agency (EMEA) made it very clear in their position statement that therapies made from both compensated and non-compensated donors are safe [3].

During my visits to plasma collection centres, I speak to donors to learn about their motives, but also to say thank you and express my appreciation. It is a good human action that deserves our utmost respect. I have seen donors who changed from being a blood donor to a plasma donor. Has this donor now become a bad donor because a reasonable compensation is given for their time and efforts? Of course not; I believe one should have the greatest respect for a person who is willing to donate plasma in a greater frequency and volume compared with a blood donor! Ethical specialists have stated that it is important that there is no undue inducement, which could happen when a compensation might be outrageous. With the average compensation that plasma donors receive this is not the case.

It is unethical not to do everything we can as a society to collect blood and plasma for the so badly needed therapies. It is my view that it is also unethical not to have measures in place to collect sufficient plasma, including compensation for time and efforts.

Safety

The manufacture of safe and effective plasma-derived medicinal products starts with the plasma collected. As mentioned above, an individual who wants to become a plasma donor has to undergo two sets of screening before being accepted as a Qualified Donor. And then, only plasma units collected from Qualified Donors that test negative for HIV, HBV and HCV are accepted.

Once collected, the plasma is kept in inventory for a minimum of 60 days before release for manufacture. This inventory holding period allows for tracing the unit in case post-donation information becomes available that would disqualify the donor (e.g. an unreported illness). The plasma that enters the manufacturing pool is extremely safe. There have been no reports of viral transmission through plasma-derived medicinal products in the last decade, proof of the robustness of the entire manufacturing process.

In contrast to plasma-derived medicinal therapies that undergo many manufacturing steps, whole blood for transfusion purposes carries a higher risk of transmitting pathogens, especially when the donations are given in the window period. Every year reports appear of viral transmission through transfusion products [4]. Safety can only come when all parts of the system work. Safety is the sum of all measures and not the result of one step.

A recent publication of Van der Poel [5] lists a whole series of old data that are analysed over-and-over again about the question whether donor compensation is still a risk. In a published response we stated that there is no evidence from clinical studies and pharmaco-vigilance data that donor compensation increases the risk of viral transmission via plasma-derived medicinal products, which have been subject to proper screening at donation and a validated viral inactivation/removal step [6]. It is more important to focus on what can be done to improve a system instead of reanalysing old data. I am proud to be working for an Industry that takes its role so seriously by developing and implementing voluntary standards and certification programmes that have contributed to the situation that one can say that products have never been safer than they are today. The already-mentioned EMEA position statement confirms the safety and quality of the therapies manufactured today [3].

What is left is the calculation of the residual risk that an infectious unit which escaped detection (window period) enters the manufacturing pool. The findings of Dr. Schreiber comparing pools made from compensated donations and from recovered plasma show that the (theoretical) residual risk calculation show that all products are equally safe [1]. That is a comforting message for all users.

References

1 Schreiber G: Relative safety of Recovered versus Source Plasma, ISBT Vancouver, 2002.

2 Simon TL: Where have all the donors gone? A personal reflection on the crisis in America's volunteer blood program. Transfusion 2003; 43: 273-279.

3 EMEA/CPMP/BWP: Position Statement: Non-Remunerated and Remunerated Donors: Safety and Supply of Plasma Derived Medicinal Products, London, CPMP, 2002.

4 WHO: Epidemiological Fact Sheet: 2002 Update Geneva, World Health Organization, 2002.

5 Van der Poel Cl et al: Paying for blood donations: still a risk? Vox Sanguinis 2003; 83: 285-293.

6 Bult JM: Response to the review 'Paying blood donations, still a risk? Vox Sanguinis 2003; 85: 48.

J.M. Bult, Plasma Protein Therapeutics Association (PPTA), 147 Old Solomons Island Rd, Annapolis, MD 21401, USA.
E-mail: jbult@pptaglobal.org

Vyas GN, Williams AE (eds): Advances in Transfusion Safety.
Dev Biol (Basel). Basel, Karger, 2005, vol 120, p 119.

SESSION IX

Panel and Open Discussion

Moderator: *L.A. Chambers*

Vyas GN, Williams AE (eds): Advances in Transfusion Safety.
Dev Biol (Basel). Basel, Karger, 2005, vol 120, pp 121-122.

What is the Role for the Use of Incentives, Including Paid Donations?

Moderator: *L.A. Chambers*

Panelists: *C. Van der Poel, N. Mikkelsen, T.L. Simon, V. Kretschmer*

Panel proceedings summarized by *A.E. Williams*

Question posed to the panel by Dr. Chambers:

"In the past when I have asked why payment for donation influences marker rates, the first answer that most people will offer to you is that it alters donor motivation, and perhaps interferes with the accuracy of the health history. It is also suggested that payment changes the type of people that come through the door to join the programme.

What do you think it is about the payment that would result in there being a difference in the infectious disease risk among donors?"

Maintenance of an adequate and safe blood and plasma supply is a pervasive challenge throughout the world. In the absence of strong public education and appropriate social networks, the sole alternative to a non-existent blood supply is dependence on paid donation and mandated pre-deposit or replacement of transfused units by friends and family of the transfused patient. In underdeveloped countries where parentally transmitted infections are common and testing may be limited, there appears to be little argument that the most appropriate infrastructure is one that strongly urges voluntary non-remunerated donation.

Panelists generally agreed that while the historical literature in the developed world convincingly shows higher rates of infectious disease markers and potential for infectious disease transmission from paid donors (both whole blood and plasma), the situation in today's well-controlled collection environment is not quite so straightforward. Under carefully defined conditions, recent evidence has shown that the marker prevalence of test results for paid collections can be equivalent or lower than the prevalence for voluntary donations. Examples of this include use of well-characterized repeat donors for paid platelet apheresis, use of an older female population for collection of anti-D plasma, and the use of strict prequalification criteria for paid plasma donors.

Disagreement also exists about the proper definition of a "paid" donation. An accurate donor screening history is likely to remain suspect among potential donors for whom payment for donation is either of extreme importance, or has become part of a donor's anticipated income stream. However, several panelists challenged the current U.S. FDA distinction between cash (or something of material value that is readily convertible to cash) and a recognition award that is not cash convertible. It was argued that everyone donates blood or plasma "for a reason" and one person's need to express themselves through altruism resulting in a donor pin, may be a stronger motivational influence than a travel or parking reimbursement to someone who does not really need a small sum of money.

In the U.S., whole blood collections are now exclusively voluntary and source plasma collections (which require a more extensive time commitment) are mostly paid. In both situations, known associations between infectious disease risk and donor demographics has led to disproportional collection volumes in the more rural geographical areas of the country (particularly the Midwest), and at college campuses.

While two distinct systems (voluntary whole blood donation and paid source plasma donation) co-exist relatively quiescently in the U.S. the same is not necessarily true in Europe and elsewhere. Where paid and non-paid systems compete with one another, numerous social and ethical difficulties arise. Payment will most certainly attract some individuals who would otherwise participate as qualified voluntary donors. However, the possible deterioration of co-existing voluntary systems by the presence of a paid donation option may be more extensive. A recent publication of survey research from the National Heart, Lung, and Blood Study REDS study in the U.S. showed that when cash-equivalent rewards are offered for donation, there are segments of the voluntary donating population who may be offended and cease their long-term patterns of voluntary donation.

A variety of donation systems were described in the panel discussions, including the strictly all-voluntary systems of Canada, the U.K., Finland, and the Netherlands. These were contrasted with payment of qualified donors in other parts of Europe, including a partially merged whole blood/apheresis plasma collection system in some parts of Germany. Sweden was described as having a paid donor system. Similarly, Norway was described as having a system where donors received gifts, which you could then have transferred into money if they did not like the gift. Despite these incentives, neither of the two countries appears to have enough donors.

The general sense of the panel was that the donor base everywhere remained fragile. Increasingly sophisticated programmes of donor recruitment, including public education and marketing, are becoming necessary components of whole blood sufficiency in an all-voluntary system. There was also concern expressed about the stability of the current voluntary structure in the face of possible future developments, such as the implementation of vCJD screening in the U.K.

Educational programmes delivered to the public about the need for blood are a critical aspect of the recruitment process. Education appears to be particularly useful when targeted to schoolchildren who are too young to donate, but are receptive to the message of social responsibility. As donation alternatives become increasingly more sophisticated to include various apheresis options, the need for qualified and committed long-term committed donors will become even more evident.

Vyas GN, Williams AE (eds): Advances in Transfusion Safety.
Dev Biol (Basel). Basel, Karger, 2005, vol 120, p 123.

SESSION X

Donor Management in the Development World: Challenges and Solutions

Moderator: *J.-P. Allain*

Vyas GN, Williams AE (eds): Advances in Transfusion Safety.
Dev Biol (Basel). Basel, Karger, 2005, vol 120, pp 125-130.

Donor Management in a Teaching Hospital Blood Bank in West Africa

J.-P. Allain[1], S. Owusu-Ofori[2], G. Bedu-Addo[2]

[1] Division of Transfusion Medicine, Department of Haematology, University of Cambridge, Cambridge, U.K.

[2] Transfusion Medicine Unit and Department of Medicine, Komfo Anokye Teaching Hospital, Kumasi, Ghana

Introduction

Blood banking in Sub-Saharan Africa is dominated by an insufficient blood supply. Most countries collect fewer than five donations per 1,000 inhabitants. This shortage leads to considerable restrictions in blood usage with the trigger for red cell transfusion often set at 4 or 5g/dl of haemoglobin. Increasing the blood supply relies on recruiting more donors, particularly volunteer donors who are in general younger and at considerably lower risk of viral infections than the older and higher risk 'replacement' donors. Replacement donors are those accepting to be bled to replace the blood transfused to one of their relatives in hospital. Replacement donations also have the financial advantage of families paying less for the transfused blood. Paid, semi-professional donors, the highest risk group, still constitute a substantial part of the blood supply in many African countries. Increasing voluntary blood collection is the main objective of Sub-Saharan Africa blood services.

Second to supply is the safety of the collected blood [1]. Depending on the country, some or all three viral markers (HBsAg, anti-HIV and anti-HCV) are tested. Full testing is performed in less than 50 % of the collected blood. Anti-HIV is screened in nearly 100 % collected units, HBsAg in over 80 % and anti-HCV in less than 50 %. The reasons for that situation are multiple and include the cost of tests (anti-HIV is still dependent on foreign aid), the belief that since HBV infection is widely spread, the clinical need for screening is minimum and the lower pathogenicity and prevalence as well as high cost of anti-HCV, often prevent the screening of blood for this marker. Added to the lack of availability of screening tests is the dispersion of blood collection and testing in hospitals collecting fewer than 1000 units per year. In this type of setting, the recommended enzyme immuno-assay testing post-donation using classical microtitre plate systems is impractical for a few samples a day and requires expensive equipment that cannot be easily maintained. The national blood service organization recommended by WHO and supported by a variety of Western aid agencies or blood services would consist of large blood centres set up according to the Western standards of collecting and distributing blood across large areas is defeated by the field reality. Even large cities do not have large numbers of donors available, communications are difficult, particularly during the rainy season, and conditions of transport (particularly refrigeration) are far from being technically feasible. Therefore, until the background situation improves, localized, small blood transfusion units based in hospitals remain the most frequent situation and solutions to ensure and maintain blood safety need to be developed and implemented. These solutions need to take into consideration local conditions, which are: (i) blood needs to be affordable for families whose average income is less than $1000, often < $500 per annum; (ii) the epidemiology is such that, in most areas, over 20 % of collected blood contain viral markers and need to be eliminated; (iii) only relatively large blood banks established in large urban areas can develop volunteer donor programmes, while the others will continue to rely on replacement blood; (iv) even if screening tests are available at a given time, sustainability of the supply is always problematic when originating from government or external aid.

Considering the extreme diversity of situations, we have concentrated this presentation on the situation of Ghana and our own blood bank established in a large Teaching Hospital in Kumasi. Practical details in an example situation might be more informative than generalization.

Transfusion Organization in Ghana

Ghana is divided into 10 regions, each of them having a regional blood bank. The Blood Service in the capital Accra collects approximately 25,000 units per year and 40 % of the donations come from volunteer donors. The Transfusion Medicine unit (TMU) in Kumasi serves a city of 1.2m. inhabitants in a 1,200 bed hospital and collected 8,000 units from 10,000 donors (50 % volunteer) in 2002. Other regional blood banks collected between 700 and 5,000 units in 2001, less than 10 % of the donors being volunteers. In addition to the 50,000 units collected annually in the main blood centres, a relatively large number of district and private hospitals collect fewer than 1,000, and often fewer than 500 units/y from replacement donors. The total Ghanaian blood supply can be estimated at around 60,000 units/y or 1.3 units per 1,000 inhabitants.

Regional blood centres, except Kumasi, which is managed by the Teaching Hospital, are managed by the Ministry of Health which has designed a national blood policy, established guidelines in blood banking, provides a degree of quality assurance and supplies blood bags and anti-HIV kits. District hospitals follow the national guidelines in blood banking. Some private hospitals are supplied with blood from the regional centres, so indirectly comply with the national guidelines, but some are collecting blood without being officially regulated. Anti-HIV is screened with different brands of microtitre EIAs or rapid tests depending on short-term contracts and external aids. HBsAg screening is performed with low sensitivity agglutination assays supplied by the individual hospitals where blood banks are located, except in Kumasi and recently in Accra where a more sensitive dipstick is in routine use [1]. Anti-HCV has been screened in Kumasi since 2001 and was recently implemented in all regional blood banks.

The Transfusion Medicine Unit (TMU) in Kumasi occupies 0.5 % of the hospital floor space and employs 17 staff members: one physician heading the unit, six laboratory technicians including one at MSc level, seven nurses (two of them trained in donor counselling), three donor organizers for the recruitment of volunteer donors, and two ancillary workers. One hospital van is essentially, but not exclusively, dedicated to mobile blood collection sessions. Since 2000, the budget has increased from $60,000 to 80,000 along with the collection of 6 to 8,000 blood units for clinical use. Whole blood or plasma-depleted red cell concentrates are used for the treatment of anaemia when haemoglobin is below or equal to 5g/dl in paediatrics (45 %), obstetrics and gynaecology (25 %), surgery (20 %) and medicine (10 %). Patients presenting with symptoms of anaemia despite a haemoglobin level above 5g/dl are also transfused. Less than 10 % of the blood supply is distributed to other local hospitals.

Blood Donor Management

Until 1997, most blood donations in the Komfo Anokye Teaching hospital in Kumasi came from replacement blood donors. Since that time, volunteer blood donors have been actively recruited and the proportion of volunteer donations has progressively and steadily increased to 53 % in 2002. Volunteer donors are essentially recruited in secondary schools that are numerous, since over 50 % of the Ghanaian population is less than 18 years of age. Secondary school students are 16 to 20 years of age and eager to help patients by giving their blood. In some schools, up to 50 % of students present to the mobile blood drives organized once or twice a year in their schools. A range of 30 to 120 units is collected in public and confessional Christian or Muslim schools per session. Through contacts with the principals and natural science teachers, donor organizers visit each school a few days before the drive date to inform students about blood and blood transfusion. They are informed that blood testing for haemoglobin level and three viral markers including HIV will be performed and that deferred donors will have the option of entering the blood transfusion donor care programme. Incentives are limited to being given notebooks, a ball pen and plastic carrier bag. In addition, a donor card will be prepared and distributed through the schools to the students. A donor card entitles the holder to a free unit for him/herself and a 50 % discount on the price of a blood transfusion required by any member of his/her direct family.

Outside the school terms, voluntary donor recruitment is more difficult. There are few large industrial companies or administrative organisations in Kumasi. However, people assemble at least once weekly in the many churches of various Christian denominations. Through contacts with the ecclesiastical hierarchy, instructions are given to the priests of the main congregations or arrangements are made with the pastor of smaller religious communities. Blood drives are organized during weekends at the outset of assemblies. This volunteer donor population is older than the secondary school students (comparable to replacement donors, median age 30) and fewer are willing to donate (range 5-30).

As a result of blood collection in schools, a blood supply of 150 to 250 units is available for clinical use during school terms but only 10 to 120 outside term. Maintaining the blood supply during these periods is the main challenge for the TMU. Since communication by post or telephone is not available, calling on donors individually cannot be done. In contrast, a large proportion of the population listens to the radio at home, at work or in the streets. We have taken advantage of this situation by establishing a close collaboration with a local FM station broadcasting in both English and the local language. Three times a year (Easter, during the summer holiday and Christmas), a blood drive located at the FM station is advertised during the preceding week. The station provides tents, sodas and T-shirts in addition to music. In the past three years, 150 to 250 units have been collected at each drive (Fig. 1). Interestingly, over this period of time, spontaneously, the percentage of repeat donors has increased from 10 to 70 %, suggesting the possibility of creating a pool of repeat donors if a line of communication is established.

In 2002, an average of 141 units/week were collected (range 50-350) or 20/day, half from replacement, half from volunteer donors (Fig. 1).

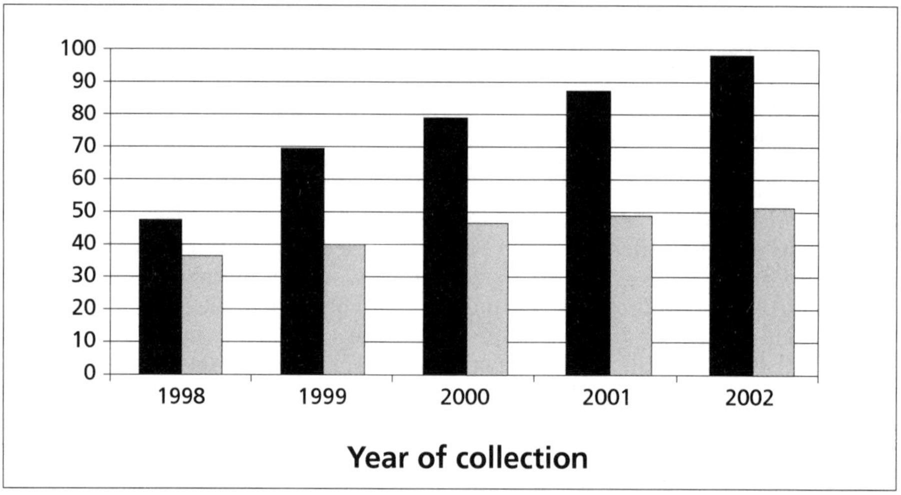

Fig. 1: Number of donors processed ■ and per cent of volunteer donors □.

IMPROVING BLOOD SAFETY WITHOUT FINANCIAL OVERBURDENING OF PATIENTS

Until 2000, blood virology screening was performed post-donation for HBsAg by an agglutination test (sensitivity 30ng/ml) and anti-HIV by an EIA test provided by the Ministry of Health. HBsAg was screened pre-donation only in replacement donors. A unit of blood was charged \$6 to families although the real cost was \$10. Families providing a replacement donation were charged \$2.5 as a processing fee. As soon as the actual costing was determined, the charges were re-adjusted to \$10 and \$4.5 for the processing fee. Given these fixed prices, considered a ceiling over which families could no longer afford transfusion, a strategy to improve blood bank efficiency and blood safety was designed. Economic studies revealed that 35 % of the TMU budget was devoted to blood bag supply, while staff salaries accounted for only 13 % of the total budget. In 2000 and 2001, three HIV transmissions had been recorded following the emergency supply of untested blood during school recesses when the blood stock was below 10 units. When blood testing was performed post-donation, the inability to communicate with deferred donors prevented them from being informed of their condition and the absence of computerized records from deleting viral marker carriers from the repeat donor panel.

To address all these issues, a strategy of pre-donation screening for all donors was progressively put into place, as previously described [2]. The initial steps consisted of evaluating the performance of various rapid tests in a dipstick format using undiluted serum or plasma. Ultimately, the Abbott 'Determine' assays for HBsAg (1ng/ml sensitivity) and anti-HIV were selected for sensitivity and specificity as well as an anti-HCV test manufactured in and distributed from China (Table 1) [2]. All three assays were purchased by the hospital for \$2.5/donor. The screening was performed from a 3ml venous blood sample enabling the Hb level as well as virological markers to be screened for in fewer than 30 minutes. This caused a slight delay in the flow of volunteers during mobile blood drives but was compatible with retention of donors. The confidentiality of screening was maintained by isolating the testing area from the donors and by delivering a neutral message of deferral without mention of the specific reactive test. Deferred donors were invited to attend the blood centre at least seven days post-deferral to perform confirmatory assays by EIA and ALT level testing for samples reactive with hepatitis virus markers. Deferred donors who attended (approximately 60 %) were given the test result, appropriate information sheet, counselling, free clinical examination and referral to appropriate clinicians in the hospital as indicated [3]. Deferred donors were not given donor cards, preventing them from entering the repeat donor pool.

As a result of the pre-donation strategy, 6 % of the budget was saved by avoiding wasting blood bags; the cost of HBsAg testing was reduced from \$1.3 to 0.75 since the testing of undiluted and 1:40 diluted sample required by agglutination tests was no longer necessary. These savings were sufficient to allow the purchase of both anti-HIV and anti-HCV rapid tests [3].

In the volunteer donor population, the deferral of sero-positive candidate donors progressively reduced the prevalence of HBsAg from 13 to 8 %. All the blood collected was suitable for clinical use and no HIV transmission occurred. Verification of the blood safety is currently being conducted using an HCV/HIV/HBV triplex applied to pools of 10 plasma samples from sero-negative blood units. The rate of

Table 1: Evaluation of rapid tests used in the pre-donation screening programme.

Marker	No samples tested	Specificity %	Sensitivity %
HBsAg	7,649	99.6	94.4
Anti-HIV	3879	98.6	100
Anti-HCV	7774	99.4	54.5*

* 95 % of the HCV RNA positive samples are detected.
Results are given compared to standard enzyme immunoassays.

confirmation for serological viral markers was approximately 99.8, 65 and 46 % for HBsAg, anti-HIV and anti-HCV, respectively (Table 1). All candidate donors with confirmed HIV positive results who attended the donor care programme (104/174) were informed, counselled and referred to the hospital AIDS clinic for follow-up. 752/1274 persons with chronic HBV infection were informed and counselled; 92 (12.2 %) had elevated ALT levels and 22 with ALT > 80IU/L (twice upper normal level) were referred to the internal medicine consultant.

Despite the relative inconvenience of slowing down the blood collection flow in mobile sessions and informing the candidate donors that they would be tested and deferred for viral marker reactivity including HIV, the number of volunteer donors kept increasing by 15 % in 2002 over the preceding year. People did not react negatively to being tested for HIV among other markers in a relatively open setting and took the donor care programme very positively.

Conclusion

Donor management in Sub-Saharan Africa needs to respond to two imperatives: supply and safety of blood at affordable cost for patients who live with less than $2 per day. The blood traditionally obtained from replacement donors needs to be substantially supplemented by volunteer donors who tend to be at significantly lower risk of carrying chronic viral infections. According to local situations, various schemes can be put in place to attract and retain volunteer donors. Secondary school students are the preferred targets in countries where a majority of the population is below 18 and the HIV prevalence still low. However, maintaining adequate blood supply when schools are closed is challenging. Strategies for blood testing should also be flexible according to local settings. National or large city blood centres may benefit from Western-type approaches using high throughput and automated methods. In the most frequent hospital settings where a small number of units are collected daily, more labour-intensive but more flexible and efficient testing strategies using rapid tests can be considered. Where the cumulative prevalence of viral markers is high (>10%), pre-donation screening may be envisaged to prepare safer blood at a lower cost.

References

1 Moore A, Herrera G, Nyamongo J, Lackritz E, Granade T, Nahlen B, Oloo A, Opondo G, Muga R, Janssen R: Estimated risk of HIV transmission by blood transfusion in Kenya. Lancet. 2001; 358 (9282): 657-660.

2 Allain JP, Candotti D, Soldan K, Sarkodie F, Phelps B, Giachetti C, Shyamala V, Yeboah F, Anokwa M, Owusu-Ofori S, Opare-Sem O: The risk of hepatitis B virus infection by transfusion in Kumasi, Ghana. Blood 2003; 101: 2419-2425.

3 Opare-Sem O, Owusu-Ofori S, Allain J-P: Novel approach to blood safety: pre-donation screening of blood donors for viral markers. Africa Sanguine Journal 2002; 5:12-16.

Professor J.-P. Allain, Cambridge Blood Centre, Long Road, Cambridge CB2 2PT, U.K.
E-mail: jpa1000@cam.ac.uk

Vyas GN, Williams AE (eds): Advances in Transfusion Safety.
Dev Biol (Basel). Basel, Karger, 2005, vol 120, pp 131-137.

Donor Management: Malaysia and the Western Pacific Region

Yasmin Ayob

National Blood Centre, Kuala Lumpur, Malaysia

Key word: Blood donors, replacement, safety, quality, organization, education

INTRODUCTION

A modern health service relies on a blood supply being available at all times. The blood service within countries in whatever form should supply safe, adequate blood and its services must be reliable, appropriate and consistent.

The Western Pacific Region is made up of countries with different cultures, languages and economies. There are well developed countries such as Japan, Australia, New Zealand and there are others that are less developed and at different phases of development. This diversity is also reflected in the development of the transfusion services. The majority are extensions of and within the context of the laboratory. Being hospital-based, these blood banks provide various services which include collection, testing, processing and issuing of blood to patients.

BLOOD DONORS

Countries in the region such as Australia, Japan, Hong Kong & New Zealand have entirely voluntary non- remunerated blood donors. There are countries where family replacement donation makes up between 30 – 100 % of the total blood supply [1] and there are also countries that recognize paid donations. In the family replacement system there may be hidden costs that do not appear within the system but are actually borne by the family. This cost may sometimes be more than in a system where the organization itself pays donors at a standard rate. The disadvantages of these two types of donors are many. These include uncertainty in terms of supply, safety and quality.

Replacement Donors

The dependency on replacement donations to supply blood is due to the fact that there is no emphasis on donor recruitment and selection. Being part of a laboratory or pathology service, it is easier to depend on replacement donors as the organization need not have the infrastructure and strategies to recruit and retain donors. It is a well known fact that replacement family donors carry a certain risk especially in terms of transfusion-transmitted disease. In certain populations the rate of hepatitis B is as high as 5-10 % which translates into 5-10 % wastage. This does not include window period donation which is more dangerous as replacement donors do not return to donate and the problem remains undetected until the recipient manifests symptoms of the disease.

The Change

The transmission of HIV through the blood supply in the early 1980s has led to considerable concern and forced countries to relook at the mechanism of the blood delivery system. It was an opportunity to reformulate policy to ensure that this virus does not contaminate the blood supply. Among the strategies employed in Malaysia are:

(i) phasing out and replacement of donors
(ii) predonation questionnaire and interview
(iii) public education through the mass media
(iv) increasing mobile clinics (paid donation did not exist in Malaysia)
(v) involvement of students in institutes of higher learning
(vi) community involvement in blood procurement
(vii) testing for transfusion-transmitted diseases
(viii) setting minimum standards and a Quality Assurance Programme

These strategies have not only improved the quality of blood donors but also the number of blood collections. Figures 1 and 2 illustrate these changes in Malaysia [2] where the number of donations increased ten-fold over three decades and replacement donors dropped from 30 % in 1980 to 1.7 % in 2002. A similar improvement is illustrated in Figures 3 and 4 for Cambodia [3]. The increase in collection is also necessary to support the ever-expanding health service as well as improvement in patient management. However, the change can take a long time, often limited by lack of financial and personnel resources. In some countries there are small communities that are remote and the need for blood is small and infrequent, so that to have excessive ready supplies of blood may not actually be economical. The need for blood for thalassemics, for example, may be required every three months and the blood group may be very specific, so that only family members can actually donate. Therefore in such instances only when blood is needed are donors called and blood collected.

Although procedures were standardized and a quality assurance programme was implemented in Blood Banks in Malaysia, there are still varying standards in donor management, processing and the use of blood. There also exist difficult communication lines between various blood banks and the National Blood Centre as the line of authority and responsibility is not direct.

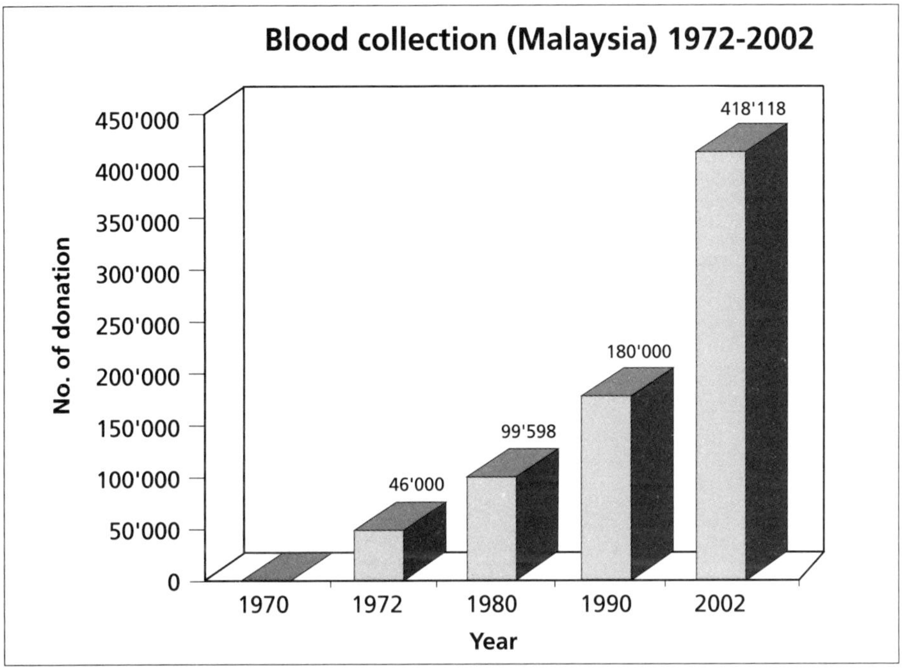

Fig. 1: A 10-fold increase in collection over three decades.

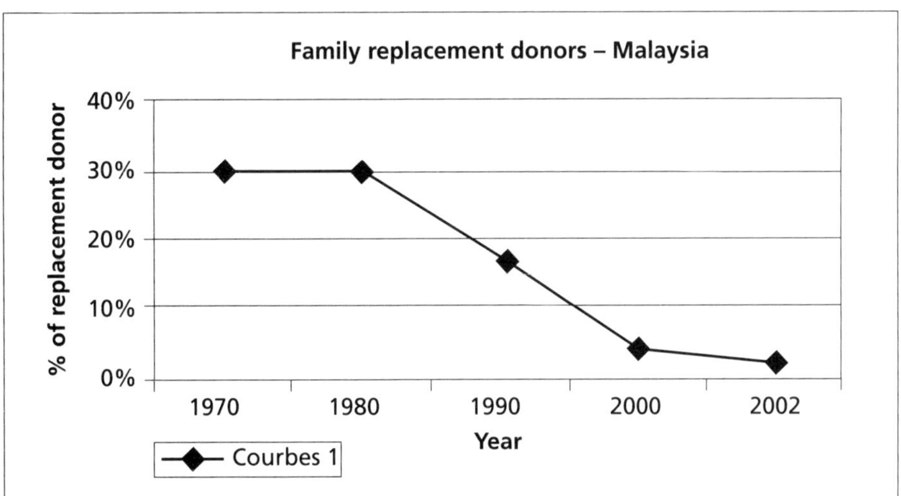

Fig. 2: A dramatic drop in replacement donors between 1980 to 2000.

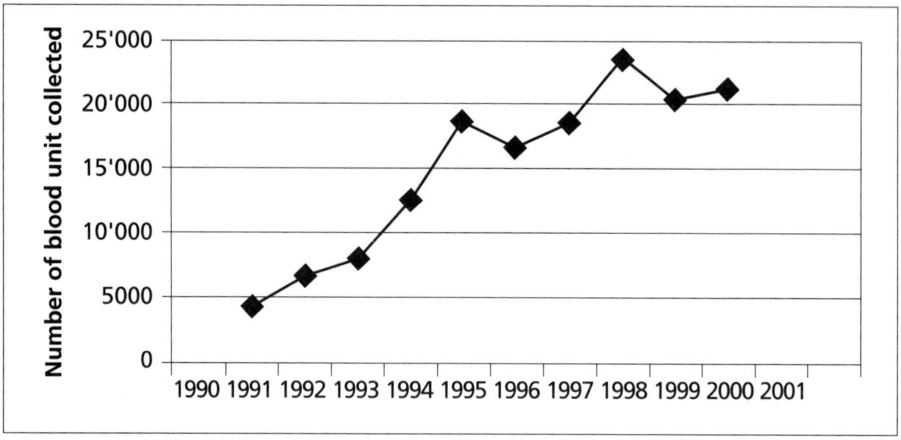

Fig. 3: Cambodia: steady increase in collection seen over a decade.

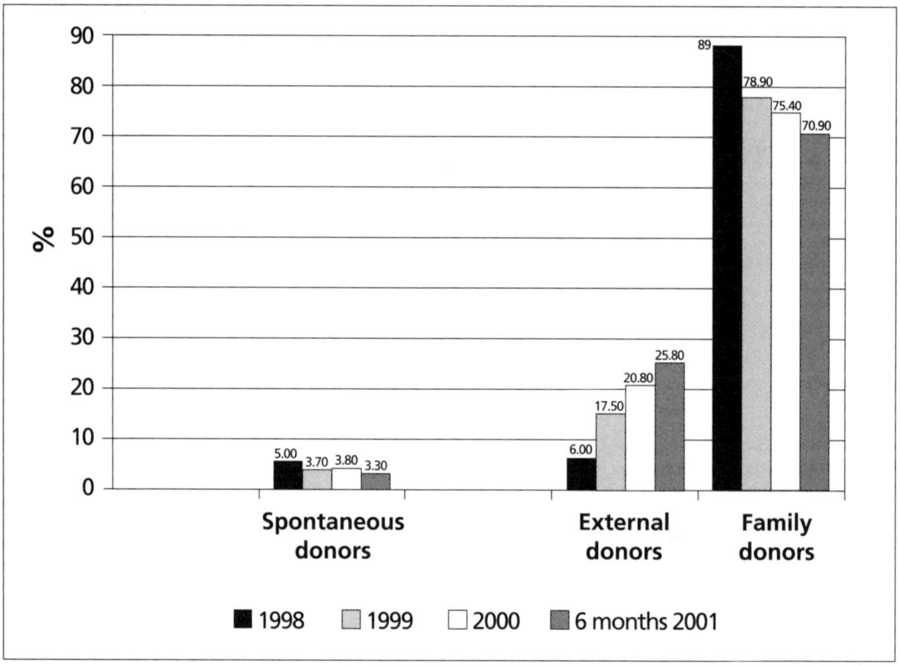

Fig. 4: Blood donors in Cambodia – External donors: donors at mobile clinics.

Hospital Base Blood Banks

As part of the laboratory services, hospital-based blood banks were able to provide fresh blood components such as red cells, platelet and plasma. However, the need for self sufficiency in blood products such as FVIII and FIX concentrate could never be achieved. This is due to lack of emphasis in donor recruitment and retention. If a department for recruitment exists it is usually poorly staffed and steps and measures to ensure a steady supply of safe blood could not be implemented. When the blood supply is low, all patients have to provide replacement donors to the blood bank before blood is provided.

There is also inefficiency within the service as there is duplication of work in common functions. There is also wastage of resources through excess processing and testing facilities. There was also variation in practice that created inefficiency, such as temporary shortage of blood resulting in rationing the supply, as it is difficult to obtain stocks from another blood bank. Alternatively some blood banks refuse to assist other blood banks in case their own supply were jeopardized.

There may also be variation in donor criteria, processing methods and test procedures. Premises for blood donation may be unsuitable and congested. Inappropriate and inadequate personnel are employed in the donor management area, resulting in poor customer service to the donors. Laboratory staff are made to process donor registration and venesection which resulted in poor donor retention.

Expertise is not developed in donor management or in other areas of the blood bank due to rotation of personnel in performing different tasks.

Progress

Recognising the weakness within the hospital system, the Ministry of Health in Malaysia is committed to the development of an integrated national service that addresses the basic requirement for national blood supplies covering safety, availability and quality. There is a need to consolidate the resources within the service and to reorganize the functional structure to ensure consistency in the quality of services provided which can be achieved through a clear line of authority and responsibility.

With the proposed organization (Fig. 5) there shall be a National Blood Centre in Kuala Lumpur and thirteen regional centres including five in the Peninsular, four in Sabah and four in Sarawak. A National Transfusion Committee shall act as a steering group to provide directional strategies for the future of the service. With this setup it is hoped that there would be an improvement in the national system through:-

(i) efficiency in donor recruitment and retention;

(ii) adequate blood collection to achieve self-sufficiency in blood and blood products;

(iii) ensure optimum use of blood;

(iv) strengthen quality system;

(v) ensure strict adherence to national guidelines by strengthening the line of accountability;

(vi) better communication between centres through electronic networking;

(vii) better management of stocks.

However, there are other shortcomings and deficiencies that would impede the process of such a development if not addressed. They include lack of transfusion specialists, lack of training for transfusion medicine in medical schools at undergraduate and postgraduate specialization level and lack of emphasis on public education.

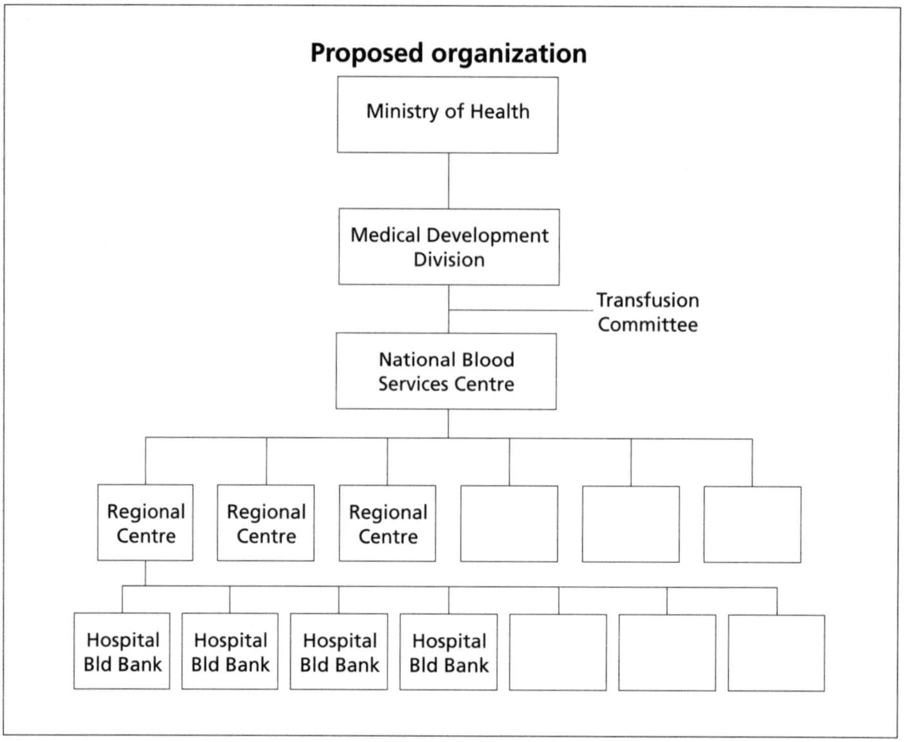

Fig. 5: Proposed organisation of Blood Donor Services.

Currently doctors who wish to specialize in transfusion medicine at Malaysian Universities would have to undergo a four-year university course for a Master's Degree in pathology. They would specialize in the sub-speciality of haematology. The course prepares doctors for diagnostic work in haematology with comparatively little exposure to transfusion. While immunohaematology and recognition of transfusion reactions are covered in the course, the candidates are not exposed to other aspects of transfusion medicine such as blood procurement, donor management, regulation control, quality management and other public health issues.

The absolute trust of patients on doctors in making decisions to transfuse relies heavily on the doctors' knowledge of the risk and benefit of blood transfusions. Doctors are ill-prepared for this huge responsibility as this area of medicine is neglected in medical school. The public is unaware of the risk and benefit. The only people who have some knowledge of this are the personnel in the blood banks and they are not involved in the decision-making. To correct this unhealthy situation both public education and training of doctors in transfusion medicine should be emphasized.

The development is also impeded by financial constraints. The service will have to compete with other medical and health-care services for usually restricted funds from the government and public. This is difficult as leaders and specialists in the field are not being trained in the most appropriate way.

Current Donor Management in Malaysia

More then 95 % of blood is collected by the Ministry of Health blood centres. More than 98 % are voluntary non-remunerated donors. Approximately 70 % are collected at mobile clinics.

Donor criteria, selection, pre-donation interview & deferral criteria are in place. However, donors with risk behaviour still donated blood. Strategies to prevent these donors from donating blood is only partially successful. At the National Blood Centre in Kuala Lumpur approximately 20 % of donors are deferred for various reasons. Fifty percent of those deferred are due to medical reasons, only 6.6 % have risk behaviour and 20 % are due to low haemoglobin levels (< 12.5g/dl).

Blood is screened for HIV, hepatitis B, C and syphilis. Approximately 2.5 % of collections are discarded annually due to the reactivity of these disease markers.

Conclusion

Blood donors are the foundation of the Blood Transfusion Service. More donors are needed each year to keep up with increasing demand from hospitals. The current donation rate in Malaysia is 20 units per 1000 population. To achieve self-sufficiency for blood and blood products the donation rate must increase one and a half times. To do this, more needs to be done to improve donor recruitment and retention. To ensure that this can be achieved, a well structured organization with a clear line of authority, responsibility and accountability should be established. Strategic direction and leadership needs to be emphasized in developing countries with appropriate staffing and funds provided. Training in appropriate areas of Transfusion Medicine with development of expertise in the different facets of this particular speciality should be a priority. It is, after all, people who make an organization work.

References

1 Chen K: Status of blood Transfusion Services in the Western Pacific Region. Report on Workshop on the Quality Management Project for Blood Transfusion Services in the Western Pacific Region (Singapore, 8 – 1 10 October 2002).

2 Blood Transfusion Service Information System. Ministry of Health Malaysia. (Annual reports 1972 – 2002).

3 Barreneche O: Country Report Cambodia. Report on Workshop on the Quality Management. Project for Blood Transfusion Services in the Western Pacific Region (Singapore, 8 – 1 10 October 2002).

Dr. Y. Ayob, National Blood Centre, Jala Tun Razak, 50400 Kuala Lumpur, Malaysia.
E-mail: yasminpd@tm.net.my

Vyas GN, Williams AE (eds): Advances in Transfusion Safety.
Dev Biol (Basel). Basel, Karger, 2005, vol 120, pp 139-144.

Taking a Closer Look at Blood Donation in Latin America

E. Vinelli

Cruz Roja Hondureña, Programa Nacional de Sangre, M.D.C. Honduras

Key words: Blood donors, socioeconomic factors, infectious diseases, demographic data, low-risk populations, safe blood transfusions.

Abstract: Shortages and unsafe blood still threaten the health of millions of individuals who need blood transfusions in Latin America. There are many demographic and socio-economical factors contributing to this situation. Poverty, high prevalence of infectious diseases, fragmented blood systems, reliance on replacement donors and hospital-based systems are undermining efforts to promote and retain voluntary non-remunerated blood donors (VNRBD) and are endangering the blood supply. Some economic factors seem unsurmountable in countries such as Haiti, Guatemala and Honduras, where the cost of processing a unit of donated blood exceeds the annual per capita budget allocation to health care. However, many countries which have chosen to coordinate their efforts nationally are able to attract 15 times more vnrbd. Working cooperatively with non-governmental agencies such as the Red Cross are also yielding higher rates of voluntary blood donors and fewer paid donors.

Shortages and unsafe blood still threaten the health of millions of individuals who need blood transfusions in Latin America. It is well known that the risk of transfusion-transmitted infections is higher when blood products come from paid or replacement donors, yet there are still countries in the region which report that 47 % of units collected came from paid donors while the majority of the blood supply still comes from replacement donors [1-2]. This article will try to address some of the demographic, cultural and economic factors affecting the recruitment and retention of voluntary non-remunerated blood donors (vnrbd) in Latin America.

The World Health Organization has stated that the pillars for a safe voluntary blood base are:

(i) nationally coordinated blood donor programme;

(ii) trained recruitment and collection staff;

(iii) donor selection, deferral, care and confidentiality;

(iv) adequate infrastructure;

(v) educational materials;

(vi) notification, counselling and referral of deferred blood donors;

(vii) collections from low risk populations [3].

We will take a closer look at each of these elements and how the countries in the region are addressing them.

If we look at the importance of a nationally coordinated blood programme we find that countries that report having such a programme or are working towards one, have on average three times fewer blood banks, collect twice the number of units per blood bank and have 15 times more units collected from voluntary non-remunerated blood donors than those countries which are not nationally coordinated (Table 1).

Table 1: National coordination, number of blood banks per country, number of blood units collected from VNRBD, number of blood units collected per blood bank and number of blood units collected per day in 18 countries in Central and South America during 2001.

Country	National coordination	Number of blood banks	Units from VNRBD	Units collected/ blood bank	Units collected/ day
Argentina	NO	752	ND	1,069	4.11
Bolivia	NO	60	2,700	412	1.59
Brazil	NO	3,000	0	588	2.26
Chile	NO	162	0	1,299	5.00
Ecuador	NO	39	23,500	1,679	6.46
Guatemala	NO	47	563	928	3.57
Panamá	NO	35	514	1,225	4.71
Average		**585**	**4,546**	**1029**	**4**
Colombia	YES	161	75,044	2,479	9.54
Costa Rica	YES	35	27,311	1,592	6.12
Cuba	YES	42	575,203	13,695	52.67
El Salvador	YES	59	7,036	1,230	4.73
Honduras	YES	29	8,378	1,268	4.88
México	YES	529	54,499	2,146	8.26
Nicaragua	YES	24	20,207	2,056	7.91
Paraguay	YES	23	1,113	2,105	8.09
Perú	YES	160	66,672	2,170	8.35
R. Dominicana	YES	81	10,153	864	3.32
Venezuela	YES	264	19,200	1,310	5.04
Average		**127.91**	**78,620**	**2810.45**	**10.81**

The Pan American Health Organization, Laboratory and Blood Services [4] are the source of data for the countries shown.

Efforts to organize the blood system and downsize the number of blood banks are definitely having a positive effect on the number of collections coming from VNR blood donors.

There is currently no information available on which countries have organized blood donor recruitment programmes, however countries that traditionally have had Red Cross involvement usually have long standing voluntary blood donor programs. If we look at Table 2, we see that countries with Red Cross involvement have higher rates of voluntary blood donors (24 % vs. 15 %) and 5 times fewer paid donors compared to countries where there is no involvement.

During 2001 the Pan American Health Organization (Laboratory and Blood Services) carried out a study to determine the knowledge, attitude and practices related to voluntary blood donation as well as the infrastructure available to service blood donors. Fifteen countries participated in this study. If we go back to the main pillars of a safe voluntary blood donor base with trained staff, informed donors, adequate infrastructure and optimal donor care, all are essential elements of this strategy. In this regard, the study found that collection staff had adequate information in terms

Table 2: Red Cross involvement, annual blood collections and percentage of paid, replacement and voluntary non-remunerated blood donors in 19 countries in Central and South America during 2001.

Country	Red Cross	Collections	% paid donors	% replacement	% VNRBD
Colombia	YES	399,171	0.00	80.00	18.80
Costa Rica	YES	55,737	0.00	51.00	49.00
Ecuador	YES	65,496	0.00	22.89	35.88
El Salvador	YES	72,545	0.00	90.00	9.70
Honduras	YES	36,781	4.83	72.13	22.78
Nicaragua	YES	49,346	0.00	59.05	40.95
Paraguay	YES	48,406	0.00	94.50	2.30
R. Dominicana	YES	70,020	2.60	82.30	14.50
Red Cross involved	**YES**	**99,688**	**0.93**	**69**	**24**
Argentina	NO	804,018	0.00	92.00	7.00
Bolivia	NO	24,747	12.55	75.68	10.92
Brazil *	NO	1,763,130	0.00	100.00	0.00
Chile	NO	210,403	0.00	100.00	0.00
Cuba	NO	575,203	0.00	0.00	100.00
Guatemala	NO	43,622	0.00	98.70	1.29
México	NO	1,135,397	0.00	95.00	4.80
Panamá	NO	42,867	47.00	51.20	1.80
Perú	NO	347,250	1.50	74.00	19.20
Uruguay	NO				
Venezuela	NO	345,953	0.00	94.48	5.55
No Red Cross involved	**NO**	**529,259**	**6.11**	**78.11**	**15.06**

The Pan American Health Organization, Laboratory and Blood Services [4] are the source of data for the number of collections and types of donors for the countries shown.

of selecting and deferring donors who had risk factors which might affect the recipient. However, they had insufficient knowledge regarding individual risk factors which might affect the donor per se. Staff reported not having enough supporting documents to carry out an appropriate interview [5].

The study also found that there was little or no consistency in the information provided to the donors [5]. This does not come as a surprise if we take into account that for 2001 the range of blood banks per country was as low as 23 (Paraguay) but as high is as 3,000 (Brazil) [4]. Transmitting a consistent message in this scenario becomes not only extremely difficult but very costly.

When donors were questioned about their experience their answers were quite revealing. They thought that blood collection sites were unattractive, uncomfortable and overall not fit for their purpose. In most cases there were no reading materials to entertain them during the waiting period and the donor interview was carried out with little privacy [5]. It is important to remember the fact that the majority of the units collected in the Region come from replacement donors and for this reason collection sites are usually located in a hospital setting, which in most cases are not the best places to provide a pleasant donor experience.

Donors expressed a clear need for more information to overcome fears and myths and would like to be reminded of the need to donate regularly, stating that they would like to receive this information first hand [5]. This is an important factor for blood programmes to take into account, especially if we take into consideration the fact that in 2001 the percentage of homes with a telephone in countries such as Honduras was only 9 %; Bolivia 17.22 %; Nicaragua 7.66 % and 13.67 % in Peru [6].

Notification and counselling of donors who have tested positive for an infectious agent are other essential elements of a safe blood donor base. There are no official reports as to how many Latin American countries actually notify donors about their serological status. It is this author's opinion that the non-availability of confirmatory tests, i.e. insufficient records that limit donor traceability and the fact that many Latin American countries have no treatment options to offer are all negative factors hindering the notification process; thus, many donors are not notified. Given the number of different blood banks in every country, a donor could easily donate again at a different site, repeating the cycle and endangering blood donor staff and possibly recipients.

How can one start to define "low-risk population"? In a continent with 48 countries and an estimated population for 2002 of 822,429,000? How and where can we find the common thread that will help us reach those groups that will provide the safest blood? Let us start by looking at how many are actually available to donate blood.

60 % of the population in Latin America is over the age of 17 and below the age of 60 [7], which are the accepted upper and lower limits for blood donation in most Latin American countries. In any given year, 2 % are women of childbearing age who will be pregnant and unable to donate blood. Since on average women are having 4.5 children [7], pregnancy and breastfeeding will usually eliminate them from the donor pool for 12 to 15 years. We should not be surprised then that 70 % of donors in Latin America are males [5].

Recent data from PAHO and the World Bank have estimated that 50 % of the population lives below the poverty level, earning less that $2 per day [7]. Since these individuals are basically trying to survive, blood donation is usually out of the question, except in those cases where blood donation is sought as a source of income. Pregnancy and poverty alone reduce the number of available donors by half.

Infectious diseases are also a major concern. In the year 2001 there were 350,000 cases of Dengue, over a million cases of malaria; between 50-60 % per 100,000 inhabitants in the Region are struggling to overcome tuberculosis and close to four million are living with HIV (Table 3). On average 4 % of donors every year will not donate again, because they have tested positive for one or more infectious disease markers, but in some countries this figure can be as high as 10 % [4].

Table 3: Total population in thousands, total number of cases of Dengue fever, total number of cases of malaria, rate of tuberculosis per 100,000 inhabitants and percentage of persons living with HIV.

Country	Total pop	Dengue	Malaria	Tuberculosis	Living HIV
Argentina	37,994	1,700	439	50-84	0.69
Bolivia	8,705	73	31,378	> 85	0.10
Brazil *	174,706	231,471	609,828	50-84	0.59
Chile	15,589	0		< 24	0.19
Colombia	43,495	22,775	107,175	50-84	0.31
Costa Rica	4,200	4,907	1,879	< 24	0.54
Cuba	11,273	138		< 24	
Ecuador	13,112	22,937	104,598	> 85	0.29
El Salvador	6,520	3,248		50-84	0.60
Guatemala	11,995	9,006	97,479	50-84	1.38
Honduras	6,732	13,642	38,143	> 85	1.92
México	101,842	21,715	7,390	25-49	0.29
Nicaragua	5,347	7,317	24,014	50-84	0.20
Panamá	2,942	317	1,036	50-84	1.54
Paraguay	5,778	24,282	6,843	50-84	0.11
Perú	26,523	3,462	68,308	> 85	0.35
R. Dominicana	8,639	21,101	697	> 85	2.80
Uruguay	3,385			25-49	0.33
Venezuela	25,093		30,320	25-49	0.49
Total no. cases	**513,870**	**388,091**	**1,129,527**		**3,648,477**

The Pan American Health Organization [7] is the source of data for the countries shown.

The economic situation of the country is another factor influencing the availability of safe voluntary blood donors. Financial resources are required to promote voluntary blood donation, screen out high-risk donors and test collections to prevent disease transmission. In the year 2000 the total allocation for health care per capita in Honduras was $52, in Guatemala $53 and in Haiti $36 [7]; the cost of collecting, testing and storing a unit of donated blood in these cases exceeds the annual per capita budget allocation to health care. In terms of availability, Cruz and Perez have reported that in Latin America the highest GNP countries have 8.5 times as much blood available per person as do the lowest GNP countries (1.79/0.21). The same study the showed a clear relation between higher GNP per capita and more VNRBD [8].

Information is a powerful tool; the combined efforts of the PAHO and national blood programme coordinators from Latin America have made it possible to receive data to support the decision-making process. We have learned that poverty, a high prevalence of infections, fragmented blood systems and reliance on replacement donors are undermining efforts to promote and retain voluntary blood donors and are endangering the blood supply, but we have also seen that countries which are coordinating efforts nationally and which are working cooperatively with non-governmental organizations such as the Red Cross are obtaining better results. The pillars proposed by the WHO for a safe blood donor base are valid.

The facts are that organisers of blood programmes need to listen to blood donors to increase their numbers, and governments need to start making the right decisions and allocating the necessary resources to obtain a blood supply that is both safe and sufficient.

References

1 International Federation of Red Cross and Red Crescent Societies: Making a Difference. Recruiting voluntary, non-remunerated blood donors. Geneva, IFRCRCS, 2002, p 15.

2 Pan American Health Organization: Report of the 124th Session of the Executive Committee. Washington, D.C., 21-25 June 1999, pp 4-5.

3 World Health Organization. Aide Memoire for National Blood Programs. Geneva, WHO, 1999.

4 Pan American Health Organization: Medicina Transfusional en América Latina. Washington, OPS/HSE-LAB/09, 2002, pp 39-47.

5 Gutierrez M, Sáenz E, Cruz J: Estudio de factores socioculturales relacionados con la donación voluntaria de sangre en las Américas. Rev Panam Salud Publica/Pan Am J Public Health 2003; 13 (2/3): 85-90.

6 International Telecommunications Union: Basic Indicators 2001. Geneva, UIT, April 2003, pp 2-3.

7 Pan American Health Organization: La Salud en las Américas. Washington, OPS, 2002, vol 1, pp 6-8, 100, 169, 332, 335, 337-9, 344.

8 Cruz J, Pérez-Rosales M: Availability, safety, and quality of blood for transfusion in the Americas. Rev Panam Salud Publica/Pan Am J Public Health 2003; 13 (2/3): 103-109.

Dr. E. Vinelli, Cruz Roja Hondureña, Programa Nacional de Sangre, 2 avenida de Comayaguela, M.D.C. Honduras.
E-mail: cenasa@honduras.cruzroja.org

Vyas GN, Williams AE (eds): Advances in Transfusion Safety.
Dev Biol (Basel). Basel, Karger, 2005, vol 120, pp 145-153.

Donor Management in South-East Asia Region (SEAR)

Z.S. Bharucha

Bombay Red Cross Blood Centre, Mumbai, India

Key words: Donor management, South-East Asia.

Abstract: Quality management of a BTS starts with safe donor recruitment and donor care. In the South-East Asia region (SEAR) almost all countries except Thailand depend heavily on replacement of blood from relatives and friends. Most of these countries except Bangla Desh have ruled out the paid-donor system; however in the guise of replacement donation it still exists. Lack of resources, lack of professional management, myths and misconceptions arising from cultural and social differences form a barrier to blood donation. Most of the countries still do not have a National Blood Policy and/or a well planned blood programme. Besides recruitment, the donor screening and donor management are also not well addressed. The donors are mainly males of 20-35 years who come from the middle class of the society. Only 3-6 % of females donate blood. Most of the donors donate once in a lifetime as there is no emphasis on retention programmes. Only 5-10 % are repeat donors. The autologous transfusions are not widely practised. However, insistence on directed donors has increased. The prevalence of transfusion-transmissible infections in the region is variable; HIV 0-1.6 %, HBV 0.06-8.5 %, HCV 1.2-3 %. Training of staff and volunteers involved in the programme has started. Countries such as India and Sri Lanka are introducing NBP and moving towards reorganisation of their blood programme. All countries have now realised a need for regulation and implementation of a quality system as well as increased their efforts towards donor recruitment and retention. To improve the safety of blood supply, all are trying to phase out the replacement system and move towards 100 % voluntary non- remunerated regular blood donation. The aim of the presentation is to highlight the problems encountered as well as strategies used in making adequate and safe blood available.

The mission of any blood transfusion service (BTS) is to provide adequate quantities of superior quality and safe blood and blood components for all in need whenever and wherever required.

Although the emergence of HIV, and other new viruses, has shifted the attention of developed countries more towards safety, the developing countries have not yet achieved adequacy. In the 10 countries of the SEA region there are 2670 blood banks which collect approximately seven million units of blood per annum [1]. A reported deficit of eight million units at times leads to mortality related to blood loss, but often results in delays in supply as well as surgeries during the seasonal shortages. In spite of a large available human resource, all these countries lag far behind in their requirement as compared to the developing countries. Table 1 shows blood collection in all SEAR countries per 1000 population.

Table 1 : Blood collection in SEAR countries.

Countries	VBD/1000 population
Bangladesh	1.75
Bhutan	2.9
India	3
Indonesia	5.1
Maldives	1.98
Myanmar	3
Nepal	2.46
Sri Lanka	7.9
Thailand	2.14

The main causes of failure of a donor recruitment programme is lack of trained staff, lack of IEC material and transport, presence of myths and misconceptions and a low rate of education and literacy. No formal training is given to the volunteers. There is no planning or scheduling of collections leading to seasonal shortages. All hospital-based centres try to carry out their own motivation and education programmes. Information provided to potential donors is not consistent and rather confusing. The donor recruitment is carried out by an outside agency and not by BTS itself and often there is no coordination and cooperation between the two, which mitigates many efforts. Very often the donor recruitment job is assigned to doctors and/or nurses working in the blood banks. Due to lack of resources, blood centres are not equipped to provide the donor services as per their expectations.

With the existing limitations and restricted resources, maximizing the safety of blood becomes a difficult task which requires a multi-layered strategy. The first essential key to the blood supply chain is **safe blood donors**. The two other important steps are **safe blood and safe transfusion practice.** Providing safe blood collected from safe donors that has undergone stringent testing with quality control measures as well as processing that ensures removal of infectious agents and/or cells faces many constraints. Safe transfusion that minimizes the unnecessary use of blood and blood components and advocates optimal clinical use of blood is not practised.

Monitoring of blood safety is easier in a centralized BTS. However in all SEAR countries the BTS is hospital-based except DPRK and to some extent in Thailand and Sri Lanka. The BTS is managed totally by the National Red Cross society in Nepal, Thailand and Indonesia and partly in India and Bangladesh. The BTS in Sri

Lanka, DPRK, Maldives and Bhutan are managed by the government. Private blood banks exist in most countries especially in Bangladesh, India and Myanmar in the region. To improve accessibility a large number of centres have mushroomed in all countries. Nearly 30 % of blood banks in the region collect fewer than 1000 units/year and this compromises cost efficiency [2]. Individual hospitals manage their own blood supplies with increasing chances that records of the total number of transfusions may be incomplete. Donor screening and blood testing procedures also vary considerably. Universal internal quality control is not implemented although the External Quality Assessment Scheme (EQAS) is to some extent introduced by WHO SEARO. Thus a significant proportion of units classified as safe even though infected may be transfused. This happens especially because of insistence on the use of whole blood, fresh blood and single unit transfusions. Five to 10 % of HIV infection in the region is transmitted through transfusions [1]. In India 78 % of HIV infection is attributed to a heterosexual mode of transmission and about 3.27 % due to blood transfusion [3].

The quality management of a blood programme starts with donor recruitment and donor care. A donor is a vital spoke in the gigantic wheel of ultimate success of the blood programme and is dependent on donor recruitment. Without blood donors there can be no blood. Without voluntary blood donors, BTS cannot ensure a supply of good quality blood in the right quantity at the right time and without donor motivation there will not be many voluntary donors. To motivate people to donate blood voluntarily is a demanding task.

People are illogical creatures often driven by emotion. They are not machines which follow commands. Their self motivation from within needs to be kindled. Knowing the potential donor is thus important for which many KABP studies have been reported. We carried out a study of public perception of blood donation jointly with the Market and Opinion Research International (MORI) which showed that important reasons for not donating blood was "not being asked" and fear of contracting AIDS through blood donation. Many in the group had not donated blood in the last three years and the chief reason for a lapsed donor was "blood was not required for a known patient". The main reason for not being a regular donor was lack of knowledge regarding the regular requirement of blood [4].

The advancement in the health care sector has increased the demand for blood; however the blood collections have not been able to keep pace. In the SEA region the collection has increased by nearly 2.2 millions since 1992 [1]. As per SEARO report, the voluntary donations have increased from 54 % in 1988 to 61 % in 1999 and the paid donors have decreased from 14-7 % [1]. Until 1999 the paid donors in Bangladesh accounted for 70 % but this was markedly reduced to 18.78 % by 2002 [5]. The number of family or replacement donors has remained static. It appears that in the absence of resources required for recruiting voluntary donors, it has been easier to get replacement donors from relatives and friends. As the system is patient-oriented, the patients and their relatives are coerced, leading to paid donors masquerading as relatives in many cases. This goes unnoticed due to the complacency of the staff as well as the authorities. In India, especially in Maharashtra a system of issuing a credit card to voluntary donors is introduced. The donors can procure a unit of blood for themselves or their relatives when in need against this card. This practice has converted many donors into depositors as they feel they have a card for their future requirements and do not need to donate again. The delay in receiving cards also affects the recruitment programme negatively. This system is also an offshoot of the patient-oriented system of blood supply. In India, the NBP approved by cabinet in 2002, has suggested moving towards 100 % voluntary blood donation and making the hospitals responsible for the blood supply and not the relatives. Table 2 shows the country-wide percentage of voluntary blood donors.

Table 2 : Country-wide percentage of voluntary blood donors.

Countries	Voluntary donors %
Bangladesh	10
Bhutan	85
India	45
Indonesia	81
Maldives	95
Myanmar	65
Nepal	92
Sri Lanka	53
Thailand	90

Many countries consider replacement donors also as voluntary donors. The percentage of voluntary donors varies depending on the efforts of donor organizations in different regions. In most countries in the region, blood collections during religious functions and in the presence of religious leaders have been very successful as the motivation level among the people attending these functions is high. Table 3 shows voluntary blood collections in different states of India in 2002.

A study done by NACO in India showed that i) 25 % of people are exposed to voluntary blood donation campaigns in different states and ii) 5 % of people had donated blood in the past year [6].

According to country reports, the 18-30 years of age group predominates among the blood donors may be because blood collections are mainly targeted in educational institutions. In India, if all attaining 18 years of age donate blood, it may just be enough but life is not always arithmetic. It is noticed that women donors donate more often between the age of 40-50 years. According to our earlier study only 12.2 % of donors were above the age of 40 years and merely 2.6 % were above 50 years [7].

The ratio of female donors in general is less as most of the country reports show only 6-8 % as female donors. The female donors predominate among the new donors enrolled as their level of motivation is higher but often deferred due to low haemoglobin and iron depletion related to menstrual loss and childbirth [8]. Very often the organizers do not approach women due to the misconception that women are weak. Some centres do report higher rates as they have introduced specific strategies to target female donors. These are as under:

- Blood collections in girls' colleges.
- Arranging family donations.

Table 3 : Voluntary blood collections in different states of India — 2002.

No.	State	% of VBD	No.	State	% of BBs
1.	Andhra Pradesh	41.1	16.	Maharashtra	79.2
2.	A & N Islands	67.6	17.	Meghalaya	1.9
3.	Assam	30.5	18.	Manipur	7.3
4.	Arunachal Pradesh	95.3	19.	Mizoram	34.5
5.	Bihar	35.8	20.	Nagaland	–
6.	Chandigarh	47.8	21.	Orissa	16.1
7.	Delhi	16.0	22.	Pondicherry	33.0
8.	Goa	37.2	23.	Punjab	14.1
9.	Gujarat	52.5	24.	Rajasthan	10.8
10.	Haryana	23.2	25.	Chennai MC	83.2
11.	Himachal Pradesh	57.9	26.	Tamil Nadu	57.3
12.	Mumbai MC	48.0	27.	Tripura	36.4
13.	Karnataka	42.3	28.	Uttar Pradesh	29.5
14.	Kerala	39.5	29.	West Bengal	80.3
15.	Mahya Pradesh	21.9	30.	Ahmedabad	53.7
					Total 45.2 %

- Donations for couples on marriage anniversaries.
- Screening by female staff.
- Use of top sheets during blood collection.

Social status and cultural differences are also noticeable in the donors and non-donors. The lower participation of some communities relates to lower education and lower income groups. In our study 76.2 % were among graduates and professionals [7]. The rich try to get blood at a price and make their employees donate blood instead.

Thalassemia is commonly seen in all countries in the region. There are nearly 30 million carriers in India and almost 10,000 are born each year. As there are many communities afflicted with thalassemia, sickle cell anemia and haemophilia, many patient advocacy groups and dedicated donor groups for specific patients have been formed. In Maharashtra state a scheme of providing free blood transfusion to these patients has been introduced.

The autologous transfusion in this region is very rare except in some major medical centres where pre-deposit, haemodilution as well as intra-operative salvage is in use [9,10].

Following many reports of high prevalence rates of transfusion-transmissible infection (TTI)s in multi-transfused patients, many patients and their doctors reeling under a loss of confidence in BTS, insist on directed donors. A case of a mother getting HIV infection from her son's blood was reported in the press from one of the states in India. The son was not able to reveal his unsafe sex practices, as he was not sure of the confidentiality of the system. Some cases of PT-GVHD have also been brought to light and have asked for legal compensations.

All countries depend mainly on first time donors. Repeat donors are generally reported as 5-10 % except for 40 % regular donors in Nepal and Sri Lanka and 50 % in Thailand [2]. Increasing efforts are now seen in many countries in the region towards improving donor recruitment and retention, such as recognition of donors and donor organizers to increase their loyalty and a number of awareness campaigns including school programmes. However there are many impediments as under:

(i) Lack of donor databases and management information systems. Computerisation of donor databases is virtually non-existent in Bangladesh, Bhutan, Maldives, Nepal and Sri Lanka. In the remaining four countries not more than 1/3 of blood centres have computerized data. In the whole SEA region only 18 % of blood banks have computer facilities [2]. Technology infusion is critical for better analysis and retrieval.

(ii) Lack of trained staff. Only 40 % of blood centres in the region have a donor recruitment officer [2]. Human resource is the backbone of the programme. Training programmes are now being conducted for donor recruitment and donor clinic staff as well as volunteers from donor organizer agencies in the region, by WHO SEARO. Short-term training courses are also being conducted by the national BTS in some of the countries. The Association of Voluntary Blood Donor Organisers (AVBDO) of Calcutta, India has a formal certificate course. Due to lack of staff and other resources, the recruitment activities are carried out by outside agencies. Often there is no coordination between BTS and the outside donor organizer agencies, causing confusion and mitigating many efforts.

(iii) Lack of material for information, education and communication (IEC). Public trust is a very fragile relationship and needs constant nurturing. Donors are blissfully unaware of the need to donate regularly. There are no sustained efforts seen in this direction. The publicity materials regarding the prevalence of transfusion-transmitted infections and their risk factors, although made available, do not match the quantity and quality required for the population.

(iv) No follow up of deferred/lapsed donors. There are no registers of such donors. Importance of these registers is now being realized.

(v) Lack of facilities for a donor-friendly environment is a major deterrent.

(vi) Lack of funds. Stable financing for blood programmes with an earmarked fund for recruitment is vital for continuous recruitment activity. The costing of services does not consider recruitment costs. Most of the programmes are run on a not-for-profit basis and hence are not well resourced. The major brunt of limited funding is always borne by the recruitment programme as other statutory requirements are a must.

In the presence of unreliable laboratory testing and a high chance of a window period, donor screening is a vital factor in blood safety. Public awareness for safe blood and transfusion-transmissible infections is increasing steadily. A baseline study of NACO reported an awareness level in India of 9-35 % in rural areas and 68-94 % in urban areas [6]. However donor selection is not rigid and self-deferral is almost absent. The donor screening procedures are not uniform and need to be improved to include the questions regarding high risk behaviour which are often not asked. Some centres do have a risk-behaviour questionnaire and some centres also have a donor unit exclusion system. Many centres do not have trained donor recruiters and counsellors and no special room to maintain confidentiality, hence no time is spent for one-to-one counselling of donors. According to a SEARO report, a private interview is not done in Bangladesh, Indonesia, Myanmar and Nepal and is only partly done by some of the blood banks in India. Maldives, Bhutan, Sri Lanka and Thailand do carry out private interviews [2]. Asking about sexual history is considered an embarrassment in most of the countries in the region. Nearly 60-80 % of blood is collected at the outdoor sessions. However, at the outdoor drives, mainly in India and Bangladesh, the organizers consider meticulous donor screening as meddlesome and unnecessary and thus quality is often compromised to achieve quantity. The informed consent is just one more signature obtained from the donor.

There have been press reports from Singapore and Australia, of donors being prosecuted and imprisoned for not having revealed their risk behaviour at the time of blood donation. It is thought to be difficult to introduce such a law in the countries in SEA where blood collection figures are so low and this punitive action might prove to act as a deterrent against recruitment efforts. However in India, under the IPC (Indian Penal Code) section 269, a donor can be held legally liable for negligent behaviour causing harm to a recipient.

According to the WHO-SEARO report, all blood units collected by the member countries are not screened for all infections. In all countries in this region, tests for anti-HIV1 & 2, HBs Ag, and syphilis are mandatory. Except for India where testing for malaria is mandatory, other countries are required to ask for a history of malaria. Anti-HCV is not yet mandatory in many countries, mainly because of high cost of the kits. It is not done in Bangladesh, Bhutan and Myanmar and partly done in DPRK, Indonesia, Maldives, Nepal and Sri Lanka. The prevalence of infections in the region is reported as: HBV – 0.06-8.5 %, HCV – 1.2-3 %, HIV 0-1.6 %, syphilis 0.5-16 % [1].

The prevalence of transfusion-transmitted infections is much less in voluntary donors compared to replacement and paid donors and in regular donors compared to first-time donors. Similar findings are reported by many centres in the region. Following a constant rise in voluntary donations, a constant decline has been reported in the HIV sero-reactivity of blood donors in Maharashtra from 1998 to 2002. The Myanmar central blood bank report shows that HIV reactivity was higher in replacement than in voluntary donors and the prevalence was reduced when the number of regular donors was higher.

For HIV reactive units almost all countries except Thailand and Sri Lanka have adopted a policy of using WHO strategy – I, whereby the reactive units are discarded and the donors are not informed as results are not confirmed. Post-donation counselling is carried out in Sri Lanka and Thailand. It is not done in Bangladesh, Bhutan and Nepal and partly done i.e. by some blood banks in Maldives, Myanmar, India and Indonesia [2]. In India following long-drawn-out ethical controversies and debates, the new plan of action has suggested implementation of post-donation information of test results after confirmation and counselling of donors, with involvement of voluntary counselling and testing centres (VCTC) in the programme. This will be an enormous task as confidentiality needs to be maintained. Once this system is in place, it will be possible to estimate risk behaviour characteristics and demographic details in these HIV-positive donors which may in turn help to formulate correct donor deferral strategies.

The following new initiatives are seen in the SEA regional countries which are likely to have an impact on the quantity and quality of blood supplies:

(i) A NBP and a plan of action for its implementation are being framed in many countries e.g. India, Myanmar, Sri Lanka etc.

(ii) Restructuring of the blood programme e.g. in Sri Lanka is reorganizing the BTS under the Japan Bank of International Cooperation (JBIC) project. In India, as recommended by the Supreme Court of India, a National Blood Transfusion Council and Blood Transfusion Councils in all states have been formulated.

(iii) For ensuring the quality and increasing cost efficiency, countries are planning the centralization of some of the activities. In India, the State Blood Transfusion councils are asked to link all the blood banks. The Drug Control Authority has permitted the establishment of storage centres to ease the access of blood in remote and rural areas. The small blood banks are also permitted storage of components from larger centres to improve the use of blood components. In Sri Lanka only six centres are planned to carry out tests for TTIs on all blood collected all over the country.

(iv) The inexorable thrust and emphasis on striving for excellence in recruitment and retention and moving towards 100 % voluntary blood donation, phasing out the replacement donors, is seen in all countries.

(v) The use of computers and information technology to assist the development of donor database and networking of blood centres is also being introduced in many countries.

In spite of all these activities, enormous challenges still remain.

Acknowledgements

Dr R. Bhatia, WHO-SEARO
Dr P. Salil, NACO, India
Dr S. Jadhav, Maharashtra, India
Dr A. Aziz, Jakarta, Indonesia
Dr M. Rajkarnikar, Khatmandu, Nepal
Dr C. Manchanayake, Colombo, Sri Lanka
Dr R. O'Chaoen, Bangkok, Thailand
Dr T. Aung, Yangon, Myanmar

References

1 Blood Transfusion Services in South-East Asia. A Status Report: WHO, SEARO, 2001.

2 Blood Centres in South-East Asia – WHO, SEARO 2003 (under printing).

3 Annual Report, NACO, India 2002.

4 Prakash Nijhara, Social Marketing – Barriers to Blood donation (Public Perceptions), in Bharucha Z (ed): Organisation and management of BTS, DTM, TMH, Bombay 1998, pp 75-78.

5 Promotion of Voluntary non-remunerative blood donation. Report of a sub-regional training course Aurangabad, WHO SEARO, 2003.

6 BSS report. NACO, India, 2001.

7 Bharucha ZS, Rajadhayaksha SB, Mangaonkar PM, Marathe SV: A study of intrinsic motivation levels in blood donors. Ind JHBT 1992; 10: 63-65.

8 Elavia AJ, Thomas A, Coyaji G: The state of women donors in Pune India A preliminary data Organisation and Management of BTS 1998; A-8: 71.

9 Ginda M, Vishwanathan C, Patil M, Rane P, Deodhar KP: Autologous Transfusion – A study of 34 cases. IJHBT 1993; 11: 152-154.

10 Bhasin R, Mahapatra AK, Banerji AK: Auto Transfusion on neurosurgical operations. J Ind Med Assoc 1993; 91: 162-163.

Dr. Z.S. Bharucha, Bombay Red Cross Blood Centre, Town Hall Compound, Shahid Bhagat Singh Road, Mumbai, 400001, India.
E-mail: zsbharucha @ rediffmail. com

Vyas GN, Williams AE (eds): Advances in Transfusion Safety.
Dev Biol (Basel). Basel, Karger, 2005, vol 120, p 155.

SESSION XI

Movement Toward International Harmonization

Moderator: *C. Smit Sibinga*

Vyas GN, Williams AE (eds): Advances in Transfusion Safety.
Dev Biol (Basel). Basel, Karger, 2005, vol 120, pp 157-163.

Movement Toward International Harmonisation. Activities of the WHO, GCBS and Council of Europe

J. Koistinen

Finnish Red Cross, Blood Service, Helsinki, Finland

Key words: International harmonisation, blood safety, WHO, GCBS, Council of Europe

INTRODUCTION

Regardless of the somewhat different explanations for the term harmonisation ("to bring into harmony" [1], "harmonise = to be or make something harmonious, harmonious = free from disagreement or ill feeling" [2]), its basic meaning is the same, to agree on matters. In blood banking this means agreement on principles and procedures of getting blood, making it into products and distributing it as well as ensuring its good quality.

The most obvious way of achieving harmonisation is by regulation and inspection. Legal power and the power of sanctions are together but one approach to harmonisation, which neither the World Health Organisation (WHO), Global Collaboration for Blood Safety (GCBS) nor the Council of Europe have. Still their work in the field of blood transfusion can improve harmonisation in transfusion medicine internationally.

The World Health Organisation is a United Nations (UN) organisation, which aims at producing health for all. Blood safety has been on its agenda for a long time, but it started receiving more attention during the outbreak of the AIDS epidemic in the middle of the eighties. With the funding of the AIDS programme a Global Blood Safety Initiative (GBSI) was started at WHO in 1988, which later led to the establishment of a unit of Blood Safety and Clinical Technology (BCT).

Global Collaboration for Blood Safety (GCBS) is an activity initiated by WHO. It is a collaborative effort of internationally recognised organisations, institutions and national representatives who are involved in improving the safety of blood transfusions.

Human rights, democracy, rule of law and social cohesion are the principles of the Council of Europe. These principles are reflected in blood transfusion as non-commercialisation of substances of human origin, voluntary, non-remunerated blood donation, self-sufficiency, and protection of donors and recipients.

Two of these, the WHO and the Council of Europe, are official inter-governmental organisations and GCBS is a global collaborative arrangement of several organisations and individuals. A review of the missions and methods of operation of these reveals how their work may contribute to international harmonisation in transfusion medicine.

World Health Organisation (WHO)

The Unit of Blood Safety and Clinical Technology (BCT) is the unit at WHO in Geneva, which carries the responsibility of promoting blood safety in that organisation. Its mission is "To promote blood safety, quality and adequacy of blood and blood products, and the selection of appropriate and cost-effective diagnostic and therapeutic procedures which are essential for the provision of healthcare" [3].

The mission fits into the four strategic directions of WHO: (i) reduction of excess mortality of poor and marginalized populations: by increasing access to safe blood, blood products, injections, clinical and diagnostic technology and medical devices; (ii) reducing the leading risk factors to human health: by creating a safe environment for the use of blood and blood products, and injections, thus reducing the risk of blood-transmissible and transfusion-related disease; (iii) developing sustainable health systems by building sustainable management capacity in the technologies involved in blood and blood products, injections, as fundamental components of sustainable health systems and (iv) developing an enabling policy and institutional environment, and promoting an effective health dimension in development policies by developing global norms and standards and, within the framework of agreed plans of action, support national policies for blood products and appropriate health technology.

The four primary objectives of the BCT relate to policy, quality and safety, and access and use of blood. Its targets relating to blood safety under these primary objectives are listed in Tables 1-3.

Table 1: The strategic targets of WHO/BCT in transfusion policy.

Target 1.	Formulation, implementation, monitoring, and updating of national policies and plans
	Advocacy for nationally co-ordinated blood transfusion programmes
	Strengthening diagnostic laboratories through appropriate national policies
Target 2.	Global collaborations
	Participation in world-wide networking through Global Collaboration for Blood Safety (GCBS)
Target 3.	Global systems to monitor impact
	Global database on blood safety

Table 2: The strategic targets of WHO/BCT in quality and safety of blood transfusion.

Target 4.	Development and establishment of norms and standards, guidelines and reference materials International Biological Reference Materials for Blood Products and Related Biologicals WHO guidelines and recommendations for the production and control of blood products and related biologicals Expert Committee on Biological Standardisation
Target 5.	Research, development, and evaluation of new technologies and methods Evaluation of HIV test kits Evaluation of saliva and whole blood tests for HIV Evaluation of test kits for the detection of hepatitis B and hepatitis C Appropriate testing technologies and strategies for Chagas, Disease Biological reference preparations for the development of diagnostic tests for transmissible spongiform encephalopathies
Target 6.	Development and implementation of national quality systems Implementation of Quality systems in blood transfusion services in all member states International and regional external quality assessment schemes (EQAS) Quality assurance of plasma-derived medicinal products and plasma fractionation activities

Table 3: The strategic targets of WHO/BCT relating to the access to and use of blood.

Access	
Target 7.	Continuous and sufficient quantities of appropriate equipment and supplies WHO bulk procurement of test kits for HIV, hepatitis B and hepatitis C Access to technology for laboratory diagnostics
Use	
Target 8.	Appropriate collection, processing, and clinical use of blood and blood products Promotion of blood donor programmes based on voluntary non-remunerated blood donors Safe blood collection systems and component production Distance learning programme for safe blood and blood products (DLP) Clinical use of blood Haemoglobin Colour Scale
Target 9.	Appropriate use of diagnostic imaging and laboratory technologies Regional external quality assessment schemes for transfusion transmissible infections (HIV, hepatitis B and hepatitis C) Development of Regional External Quality Assessment Schemes (REQAS) in Blood Group Serology Establishment of regional training centres for quality management
Target 11.	Appropriate use of devices and clinical technologies Improving blood safety by ensuring reliable and appropriate HIV testing Blood cold chain Information technology in transfusion safety Access to medical devices, R & D and technology transfer to developing countries

WHO and Harmonisation in Transfusion Medicine

The generic and specific guidance given by BCT help to improve the safety of blood transfusion. These and the external quality assurance schemes assist in reaching harmonisation. The "Requirements for the collection, processing and quality control of blood, blood components and plasma derivatives" [4] is one of the best known guidelines given by WHO which improves international standardisation. Although this guidance is not binding to the member states, and neither is it compulsory for the blood transfusion services to participate in the external quality assurance schemes (EQAS), it is nevertheless easier to convince the regulators about the appropriateness of the operation of the blood transfusion service if they are followed.

Global Collaboration for Blood Safety (GCBS)

The recommendations on the need for global attention for blood safety which were made at the Paris AIDS Summit of December 1994 were reinforced by a resolution of the World Health Assembly in 1995 (WHA 48.27). Based on this resolution WHO took up the initiative and in October 1995 the first preparatory meeting was held in Geneva for the formation of a task force for Global Collaboration for Blood Safety. The meeting involved most of the major organisations and institutions involved in the area of blood safety and it reviewed the WHO proposal and formulated recommendations for a mechanism to improve global blood safety. The first full meeting of GCBS was held in November 2000.

The mission of GCBS is to promote and strengthen international collaboration on the safety of blood products and transfusion practices. The goal is to improve collaboration among organisations, agencies and institutions involved in the safety of blood products and transfusion practices, with a view to (i) encouraging and facilitating information exchange; (ii) promoting standards, including current good manufacturing practices for blood and related products for transfusion; (iii) fostering the establishment of co-operative arrangements aimed at promoting the safety of blood donors and recipients in all countries; and (iv) promoting the safety, adequacy, quality and appropriate use of blood and blood products.

The objectives of GCBS are listed in Table 4.

Participants. Intergovernmental organisations (e.g. WHO, European Commission and Council of Europe) and many international non-governmental organisations (e.g. International Society of Blood Transfusion, International Federation of Red Cross Societies, Thalassemia International Federation, International Consortium for Blood Safety, International Federation of Blood Donor Organisations), government institutions and agencies (e.g. Food and Drug Administration, U.S.A., Therapeutic Goods Administration, Australia), international industry associations and umbrella organisations (e.g. European Plasma Fractionation Association, Plasma Protein Therapeutics Association) and WHO Collaborating Centres, participate in the work of GCBS. Regional representation, in particular from developing countries is also ensured. Experts may be invited to share information and/or to advise the GCBS. The General Meeting may invite organisations and individual experts to attend all or certain designated meetings as observers. Organisations which meet the criteria to become participants, but do not wish to do so, may at their request attend as liaison.

Table 4: The objectives of GCBS are that the participants collaborate in:

1. Facilitating progress in international consensus on essential principles of global blood safety;
2. Encouraging the recognition and establishment of national blood programmes;
3. Identifying priorities for the prevention of transfusion related disease;
4. Implementation of appropriate and recognised transfusion practices, which ensure donor and recipient safety and are free from discrimination;
5. Effective recruitment of safe donors through the use of appropriate selection criteria;
6. Assuring quality and safety in the preparation of blood and blood products;
7. Safe international practices for the collection, storage and transport of plasma and the preparation and distribution of its derivatives;
8. The bi-directional traceability of blood products between donor and recipient whether in-country or across national borders;
9. Promoting evidence-based use of blood and blood products;
10. The exchange and use of information by encouraging data collection, management and dissemination.

The General Meeting of GCBS is held at least once a year and is attended by one representative from each participating organisation. It reviews activities and proposals presented by the Planning Group and recommends their content for endorsement by the GCBS participants. The Meeting selects a maximum of 12 participants for a three-year term to the Planning Group, in addition to the GCBS Chair and Vice-chair and WHO as ex-officio participants. It puts forward proposals and recommendations to the GCBS participants, accepts new participants, experts and liaisons, and establishes Working Groups.

Working groups. GCBS may establish Working Groups to address and advice GCBS on specific issues which are related to the safety of blood products and transfusion practices. Each Working Group prepares a report on the outcome of its work and presents it to the General Meeting through the Planning Group.

Although the activities of GCBS do not produce regulations to enforce harmonisation, it is reasonable to say that achievement of its goals and objectives supports harmonisation in transfusion medicine.

Council of Europe

The Council of Europe was founded in 1949 and has 44 member states. Its headquarters are in Strasbourg, France. Its principles are human rights, democracy, rule of law, and social cohesion. The principles which deal with blood are non-commercialisation of substances of human origin, voluntary, non-remunerated blood donation, self-sufficiency, and protection of donors and recipients.

Studying the ethical, legal and organisational aspects of blood transfusion, ensuring the quality and availability of blood, avoiding wastage by ensuring optimal use of blood components, and analysing the possible ethical and organisational impact of new scientific developments are the objectives related to blood.

The work on blood transfusion is done by the Committee on Blood Transfusion and Immuno-haematology (SP-HM) and the Select Committee of Experts on Quality Assurance in Blood Transfusion Services (SP-G-RS). Their work is approved by the European Health Committee (CDSP) and Committee of Ministers.

The most important work produced by the Council of Europe in blood transfusion is the so-called Guidebook, "Guide to the Preparation, Use and Quality Assurance of Blood Components", which is revised annually. Its 11th Edition was published in 2005 [5].

"The Guide" has become the accepted basic standard in Europe and many other countries, such as Australia and New Zealand. It gives standards on blood and blood components as well as guidance on donor selection, blood collection, technical procedures and transfusion practices. The standards of blood components are the most useful part of the "Guide". Upon development of new methods, material and supplies, the standards are revised annually to include the development of new methods, material and supplies. "The Guide" is not a legally binding regulation, unless national regulators, as many do, indicate that it must be followed.

Council of Europe and harmonisation. The ethical principles of the Council of Europe in blood transfusion, such as non-remunerated blood donation and the standards given in the "Guide", have a long history, and have accelerated harmonisation in Europe. Many of the members of the Council of Europe expert groups, especially of the SP-R-GS, also participate in drafting the EU directives, and the Commission of the European Union is increasingly using their expertise. This collaboration between the European Union and the Council of Europe is now developing well, after the first stages of learning the principles of drafting a law and how it differs from writing guidelines.

Thus one can conclude that the Council of Europe has great influence in the standardisation of European transfusion medicine, due to its long tradition in working for the safety of blood transfusion.

Movement Towards International Harmonisation

International harmonisation is desirable because it creates trust in the blood transfusion service processes across borders. At present the blood components do not move internationally to any great extent, but plasma and plasma products do. Blood collection and component separation are essential parts in the procurement of plasma; thus harmonisation of the first stages of the whole process creates trust and improves the safety of the raw material (plasma) as well as intermediate and end-products (albumin, coagulation factors, gammaglobulin). Globalisation may increase the crossing of borders of the blood components as well. Thus harmonised procedures and methods will improve the overall safety of transfusion.

Regulation is always binding and complete internationally harmonised regulation is understandably difficult to reach. On testing for the most important transmissible infections it is easy, but on many other matters slight differences must be allowed and it must be understood that safety has still to be the same. Decisions on international harmonisation should be made by consensus and not by dictation by some national organisations. It is also necessary to accept that political decision-making is an art of compromise; strong opinions, e.g. by experts, may complicate the attempts towards harmonisation.

Summary

The World Health Organisation, Global Collaboration for Blood Safety and the Council of Europe cannot harmonise by binding regulation, but they can bring important matters to discussion. They can also give guidelines and recommendations, and work out resolutions for national ratification. All this and also the networks created by these organisations are important in improving blood safety and harmonising the policy and practices in the field of transfusion medicine.

References

1 Webster's Encyclopedic Unabridged Dictionary of the English Language. Gramercy Books, NewYork/Avenel, New Jersey, 1989.

2 Oxford Advanced Learner's Dictionary. Jonathan Crowther (ed): Oxford University Press, fifth edition, 1995.

3 Blood Safety and Clinical Technology. 2000-2003 Strategy. Department of Blood Safety and Clinical Technology, World Health Organisation, Geneva 2001, WHO/BCT/01.01.

4 Requirements for the collection, processing and quality control of blood, blood components and plasma derivatives (Requirements for Biological Substances No27, revised 1992) In: WHO Expert Committee on Biological Standardisation. Forty-third report. Geneva, World Health Organisation, 1994, Annex 2 (WHO Technical Report Series No. 840).

5 Guide to the preparation, use and quality assurance of blood components, 11th edition. Council of Europe Publishing, Strasbourg, 2005.

Professor J. Koistinen, FRC Blood Service, Kivihaantie 7, FIN-00310 Helsinki, Finland.
E-mail: jukka.koistinen@bts.redcross.fi

Vyas GN, Williams AE (eds): Advances in Transfusion Safety.
Dev Biol (Basel). Basel, Karger, 2005, vol 120, p 165.

SESSION XII

Panel and Open Discussion

Moderator: *J.S. Epstein*

Vyas GN, Williams AE (eds): Advances in Transfusion Safety.
Dev Biol (Basel). Basel, Karger, 2005, vol 120, pp 167-169.

How Do Industry and Government Approach Product Standardization?

Moderator: *J.S. Epstein*

Panelists: *A. Farrugia, T. Evers, C. Waller, G. Sher, R. Seitz*

Panel proceedings summarized by *A.E. Williams*

An introduction and three questions were posed to the panel by Dr. Epstein:

Standards in transfusion medicine primarily arise from two sources. Voluntary standards developed by industry can be developed quickly and efficiently, but lack the weight of regulatory enforcement and may be partially driven by economic factors. In contrast, government regulation imposes a minimum standard that is enforceable and thereby fosters consistency in the areas of industry that are under its jurisdiction. However, government regulation is also generally more deliberative and less responsive to change. When driven by the forces of self-determination, regulations may also be nationally or even locally unique.

International harmonization of standards and regulations is a laudable goal, but one that is difficult to achieve. In the blood arena this is largely due to the fact that the starting materials cannot be fully characterized and standardized. In the area of labile blood products, harmonization of standards is certainly desirable, but somewhat less critical than for the plasma industry, where the product stream and business dynamics are multi-national.

Questions for the panel's consideration include:

1. *What are the significant differences in the worldwide approach to blood product standardization?*
2. *Is the current balance between government regulation and voluntary industry standard setting optimal?*
3. *How can governments and industry best approach product standardization while promoting innovations in safety and efficacy?*

A detailed description was given of the recent interactions between Canadian Blood Services (the collector) and Health Canada (the regulator). Both systems were re-focused in the aftermath of the 1997 report on Canada's blood supply by the Kreever Commission. The report concluded that the Canadian regulators and the previous operator – The Canadian Red Cross - had collectively arrived at standards that were insufficient to maximize transfusion safety. Under its newly reformed systems, initial bursts of heavy regulatory oversight have gradually given way to consultative rule-making, where Health Canada sets minimum standards, but issues directives only after giving the operators an opportunity to comment on their likely impact. The CJD/BSE deferral policies - instituted in North America in 1999, 2000, and again 2001, were characterized as involving active dialogues between the operator and the regulator in Canada, including international collaboration between the North American regulators and operators. Canada also has a system of national voluntary standards for blood collection. Unlike the AABB in the U.S., however, there is no accompanying certification process.

The manufacture of products for the entire world leads to an accumulation of disparate regulations which increases costs and leads to manufacturing and distribution inefficiencies and potential shortages of products. For these reasons, the international harmonization of standards and regulations is a front-line issue for the plasmapheresis for manufacture (source plasma) industry.

In addition to its obvious benefits for efficient manufacturing, harmonized standards tend to improve product supply by opening multi-national distribution systems. The major industry umbrella organization, the Plasma Protein Therapeutics Association (PPTA International), acknowledges the major hurdles inherent to harmonization, i.e. everyone agrees that harmonization is desirable as long as it complies with their local standards. PPTA indicated that it actively solicits and carefully considers input from its international groups of patient stakeholders and intends to continue pursuing international harmonization in small meaningful steps.

Among the European community, the current European Directive was the successful result of extensive interaction between regulators and industry. Current controversies in Europe appear to be between the conflict of voluntary and required standards, in part because the European regulatory standards are targeted to be optimal (with room for some negotiation), rather than minimal and rigid.

From the regulatory viewpoint, most regulators find themselves to be in a unique public health policy position. They are responsible for balancing the science of risk against the political acceptance of that risk, without direct regard for the third element of the mix, which is the economic cost. Blood safety is a uniquely visible and sensitive topic in all three domains. The panel discussed possible regulatory fears that a large element of industry could potentially march down a standard-setting path that might be difficult for industry peers to maintain safely. The aggressive American Red Cross donor deferrals for geographical exposure to BSE earlier in this decade was offered as an example of that scenario. In this context, the audience was reminded that restrictive voluntary standards adopted by a manufacturer become a de facto local regulatory standard once they are incorporated into an approved manufacturing standard operating procedure.

Interestingly, the Council of Europe Guide, which does not yet carry the weight of law in Europe, is mandated under the Therapeutic Goods Act (TGA) in Australia as the legal standard for blood components. The TGA also mandates that plasma collection in Australia be conducted under the standards of the British Pharmacopoeia.

Other notable efforts to improve standardization in the field of blood transfusion include the WHO Expert Committee on Biological Standardization and the WHO Global Collaboration for Blood Safety (GCBS) which is working to develop minimum requirements for blood transfusion services and blood products.

Finally, it was proposed that one practical step for harmonization which could be taken internationally would be to improve the ability to trace blood and plasma by using the unique international coding system (ISBT 128) which has been available for several years.

Vyas GN, Williams AE (eds): Advances in Transfusion Safety.
Dev Biol (Basel). Basel, Karger, 2005, vol 120, p 171.

SESSION XIII

Surveillance and Management of Medical Errors: Putting Data to Use

Moderator: *R.M. Lewis*

Vyas GN, Williams AE (eds): Advances in Transfusion Safety.
Dev Biol (Basel). Basel, Karger, 2005, vol 120, pp 173-177.

Event Reporting Systems: MERS-TM, Surveillance – Seeing and Using the Data Below the Waterline

H.S. Kaplan

Department of Pathology, Columbia University, New York, NY, USA

Key words: Near misses; event reporting, recovery, alertness

Abstract: A significant variability in reporting rates, particularly of near-miss events, limits the quantitative reliability of event reporting. Organizations tend to disregard events such as near misses if they are "below the waterline", and outside their classification schemes. High reliability organizations, on the other hand, see near misses as valuable information regarding a system's weaknesses. Another value of near-miss reporting is the opportunity to study recovery factors in order to promote recovery once failure occurs. Since transfusion procedures are well-practised routines, they are often performed as automatic behaviours, vulnerable to interruption and unanticipated occurrences. Data fed back from near-miss events are a useful means of countering this, by maintaining an attitude of alertness in task performance.

Despite the potential value of event reporting systems, including the direct engagement of staff in patient safety, a significant variability in reporting rates, particularly of near-miss events, limits their quantitative reliability in surveillance systems.

In a mail survey of event reporting in hospital transfusion services [1], with more than 2,000 hospitals responding (a 63 % response rate), two-thirds of the hospitals reported capturing fewer than one event per month, while only a handful reported three or more events per month. There was no good correlation with the number of hospital beds, number of transfusions, or surgical procedures performed. This survey, carried out in 2000-1, preceded the currently proposed FDA requirements for event reporting by hospital transfusion services [2]. Regardless of compliance with the new regulations and the likely consequence of increased reporting, it is unlikely that the majority of hospital transfusion services would report the bulk of events.

More than 90 % of events recorded over a four-year period of active collection at one hospital site using the Medical Event Reporting System-Transfusion Medicine (MERS-TM) were near misses (events that were prevented from causing patient harm by a planned or unplanned barrier) [3]. Because three-quarters of these near misses were recovered before blood unit issue, they would not be captured through mandatory reporting since they were still under the control of the blood bank. In addition, in another study of safety culture and event reporting, in 53 hospitals, only 8 % of technologists consistently reported near-miss events, and 72 % did not report them at all [4]. The top four reasons that employees did not report mistakes were: (i) the error was corrected before anything bad happened; (ii) it is easier just to fix the error than to report it; (iii) the error might be written in their personnel file and (iv) they do not want to get themselves or anyone else in trouble.

Even in environments not supportive of reporting, e.g. pathological environments, that "kill the messenger" [5], people will usually happily report on equipment failures. Next they will report on events that originated in other departments. In the more supportive reporting environments, people will report on errors caused by others within their own department. Finally they will report on their own errors, and eventually on their own rule violations. If the only perceived use of reporting is for regulatory compliance, or as entries in a personnel record, it is highly unlikely that reports go beyond equipment failures or at most, the shortcomings of other departments.

People also see what they want to see [6]. Classifications trigger information processing routines for gathering information and analysing data [7]. Near misses fall into the grey zone of classification. In a high reliability organization (HRO), such as the flight deck of an aircraft carrier, which operates in a hazardous environment, a near miss is seen as a kind of failure, revealing a potential danger. In most other organizations, because there is recovery, a near miss is considered as evidence of success [6]. In an HRO they attempt to make the most of every single minor event they encounter to prevent the more significant unanticipated and harmful occurrences.

Organizational culture, fear of punishment, a lack of resources, and lack of feedback, may all discourage reporting, particularly of near misses. Another major deterrent is that organizations tend to disregard events, such as near misses, if they are outside their classification schemes. If compliance, or "ritual compliance" rather than adoption, is the primary motivation for reporting, events outside the boundaries of regulatory requirements are less likely to be seen.

Misadventures (events with patient harm) are viewed as the tip of the iceberg – easily seen above the waterline. Events in the larger, dangerous region below the waterline (near misses and events without harm) usually require increased attention for their detection. This attention is warranted because these events, far greater in number than misadventures, reflect the system's weak points, and allow an approximation of the proportion of classes of the system's failures. Also, near misses provide valuable information about human recovery – i.e. why something bad did not happen (both planned and unplanned factors).

Unfortunately, the value of identifying factors which enhance recovery, is not generally appreciated. Current emphasis is often almost exclusively on the prevention of errors. What is actually desirable is the prevention of negative consequences, not errors per se. Promoting recovery factors that contribute to complete or partial recovery once failure has occurred is consistent with the goal of preventing or reducing the negative consequences of that failure [8].

Over the last six decades, recovery and rescue have been critical factors in the improvement observed in the rate of fatalities associated with error in blood transfusion. From the 1940s until the present, fatality rates due to error have dramatically decreased from one in a thousand, to approximately one in two million transfusions. However, the current rate of ABO incompatibility is about one in 50,000 transfusions, with almost one-half of the misadventures resulting in acute haemolytic transfusion reactions [9]. There has been far less success in preventing mistransfusion than in its recovery and mitigation. The requirements for careful observation during transfusion, and a continued emphasis on rapid investigation of untoward reactions with cessation of transfusion and rapid treatment have contributed to the significant improvement in outcome.

If an error were not prevented, the next goal would be to make it detectable so that it may be identified and corrected as soon as possible. The next level of recovery would be to localize its effect and prevent harm and, if that is not achieved, at least to mitigate the harm.

Although errors are ubiquitous in complex systems, serious harm is relatively infrequent because error recovery occurs almost continuously. In a U.K. multi-centre study of paediatric arterial switch procedures, on average seven events per procedure resulted from surgical team error. One major potentially life-threatening event occurred among these seven events; however, because of recovery, there was no impact on the baseline fatality risk [10].

Where there is continual challenge to recovery, there may be an erosion of recovery capability. When stressed beyond the limits of this capacity, failure may occur [10]. This limitation is another reason for capturing information regarding near misses, even though a barrier has performed successfully.

Three key factors contribute to the likelihood of failure and an undesired outcome or "surprise": (i) criticality; (ii) degree of "hands-on" and (iii) frequency. The processes of transfusion score high in all three of these characteristics, making them quite vulnerable to surprise. Harm to patients due to mistransfusion typically arises from errors in well-learned and practised routines with little cognitive error potential. The multiple steps in transfusion, the frequency of their repetition, and usual uneventful outcome, lead to automatic behaviour. This lack of mindfulness or decrease in awareness and conscious engagement in the task at hand increases susceptibility to error when a change or interruption occurs[11].

Patient identification and sample labelling do not present a high level of cognitive challenge; the challenge is in maintaining mindfulness in their execution. Mindfulness is a qualitatively different state of alert and lively awareness [11]. A routine mindless task such as walking through a doorway undergoes a cognitive shift when a "wet floor" sign triggers a different level of awareness of contact between foot and floor. How can the same kind of lively awareness be created in the minds of hospital staff involved in routine, very frequent, hands-on critical functions of transfusion?

Following the principle that a weak signal does not necessarily warrant a weak response (Weick), even minor events well below the waterline may aid in maintaining alertness: for example, feeding back the numbers of blood components wasted on different hospital units. By treating wasted blood components as reportable events, the rate of blood units wasted in clinical care areas provides a surrogate measure of mindfulness. The units of blood wasted on a floor because of incomplete pre-transfusion procedures and delay, may reflect an environment in which blood is not handled carefully. Such delays not only lead to wastage, but have a potential for mistransfusion, since more than one patient's blood may be available for selection at the nursing station.

Wastage caused by delays due to lack of vascular access, or missing informed consent, and losses due to improper storage are some of the factors tracked and fed back to nursing in our hospital. A new transfusion request form designed in collaboration with nursing provides reminders for pre-transfusion preparation, and serves as a checklist for critical process steps in transfusion. Following the introduction of both the form and feedback regarding wastage, there was a progressive reduction in episodes of component wastage over six months, with the last four months showing a decrease in episodes (per unit transfused x 100) compared to the prior six months. [mean: 0.6 episodes (0.4-1.0 episodes) versus 2.5 episodes (2.0-3.5 episodes)].

Evidence suggesting a heightened nursing awareness of the conditions of transfusion was perhaps as important as the encouraging decrease in blood wastage. For example, nursing protocols have been rewritten to control blood components better in the operating room, and to prevent blood from being unaccounted far more rigorously after surgery.

An interesting example of the information contained within discarded units was a blood unit spiked and discarded untransfused. It was found that the unit had been checked for identity at the nursing station rather than at the bedside. Just before starting the transfusion of the spiked unit, it was recognized that the wrong patient was almost transfused. Interestingly, this event was not reported as a near miss, but "just" a discarded unit. Not only was the neutral term "discarded unit" more palatable to the reporters, the classification scheme was also much clearer than for a near miss. If, because of a near miss recovery, "the glass is considered half-full", the chance of learning something from having almost transfused the wrong patient is very unlikely.

Looking below the waterline not only provides valuable information about the patterns and causes of failure; it can provide information about the elements of recovery, as long as an organization's classification schemes support the recognition of near misses. Of equal importance in transfusion, where many procedural steps are over-learned, it can provide data necessary for reinforcing mindfulness in carrying out routine but critical tasks.

References

1 Schreiber GB, King MR, Kaplan HS, Nieva V, Sorra J, Chang DN: Error reporting in hospital transfusion medicine services: a status report. Transfusion Suppl 2001; 41: 15S.

2 FDA Docket 00N-1484, 14 March 2003. Safety Reporting Requirements for Human Drug and Biological Products; Proposed Rule.

3 Callum J et al: Experience with the medical event reporting system for transfusion medicine (MERS-TM) at three hospitals. Transfus. Apheresis Sci. 2004; 31 (2): 133-143.

4 Sorra J, Nieva V, Schreiber G, King M, Kaplan H: Safety Culture and Reporting in Hospital Transfusion Services. Transfusion Suppl 2002; 42: 137S.

5 Westrum R: Cultures with requisite imagination, in Wise J, Hopkin D (eds): Verification and validation: Human factors aspects. New York, Springer, 1993, pp 401-416.

6 Weick K, Sutcliffe K: Managing the unexpected: assuring high performance in an age of complexity. San Francisco, CA, Jossey-Bass, 2001.

7 Tamuz, M: Defining away dangers: A study in the influences of managerial cognition on information systems, in Lant TK, Shapira Z (eds): Organizational Cognition: Computation and Interpretation. Mahwah, NJ, Lawrence Erlbaum Associates, 2000, pp 157-183.

8 Van der Schaaf TW, Kanse L: Errors and error recovery, in Elzer PF, Kluwe RH, Boussoffara (eds): Human Error and System Design and Management, London, Springer Verlag, 2000, pp 27-38.

9 Linden JV, Wagner K, Voytovich AE, Sheehan J: Transfusion errors in New York State: an analysis of 10 years' experience. Transfusion 2000; 40: 1207-1213.

10 Reason J: Managing the Risks of Organizational Accidents. Ashgate, Brookfield USA, 1997.

11 Langer E: Mindfulness. Addison-Wesley, Reading, MA, 1989.

Dr. H.S. Kaplan, Department of Pathology, Columbia University, 622 West 168th Street, New York, NY 10032, USA.
E-mail: hsk18@columbia.edu

Vyas GN, Williams AE (eds): Advances in Transfusion Safety.
Dev Biol (Basel). Basel, Karger, 2005, vol 120, pp 179-187.

Surveillance of Transfusion Errors: Putting Data to Use in the U.K.

M.F. Murphy

National Blood Service, Department of Haematology, John Radcliffe Hospital, Oxford, and the University of Oxford, U.K.

Key words: Surveillance, transfusion, error, haemovigilance

Abstract: The haemovigilance system in the U.K., the Serious Hazards of Transfusion (SHOT) scheme, was established in 1996 to collect reports of major adverse events associated with the transfusion of blood components. 92 % of eligible hospitals now participate in the scheme. The number of reports has increased every year due to an increase in the most frequent reported event, which is incorrect blood transfused (IBCT). Other complications of transfusion are all represented to a varying degree, but episodes of transfusion-transmitted infection are infrequent. The SHOT scheme has made many recommendations to improve the safety of transfusion, including that further research should be carried out into information technology solutions for safer transfusion, and into new strategies for reducing bacterial contamination and transfusion-related acute lung injury (TRALI).

BACKGROUND

Haemovigilance is an essential component for improving the safety of blood transfusion. Approaches to haemovigilance vary around the world [1], but the broad aims are to collect and analyse data on the number, type and sequelae of adverse events to transfusion, and to make recommendations for improvements in transfusion safety. This review will consider the data provided by the haemovigilance system in the U.K., the Serious Hazards of Transfusion (SHOT) scheme [2,3], and how they have been put to use for improving transfusion practice.

HAEMOVIGILANCE IN THE U.K.

The SHOT scheme was established in 1996 as a voluntary, and anonymised reporting system. It published its fifth annual report in April 2002 [2]. Although it is based in a Blood Centre and is funded by the U.K. Blood Services, it is operationally independent of the U.K. Blood Services. The scheme's umbrella organisation is the Royal College of Pathologists, which is responsible for professional activities within haematology and transfusion medicine.

Mechanism of reporting and participation in the scheme

The SHOT scheme invites reports of major adverse events associated with the transfusion of blood components; the scheme does not cover complications caused by fractionated blood products. Figure 1 shows the mechanism for reporting of non-infectious incidents by a haematologist or blood bank to SHOT, using a general reporting form. The SHOT office then returns to the hospital a specific questionnaire appropriate to the incident, and analyses the returns. Infectious incidents are reported via the local Blood Centre to the Communicable Disease Surveillance Centre (CDSC).

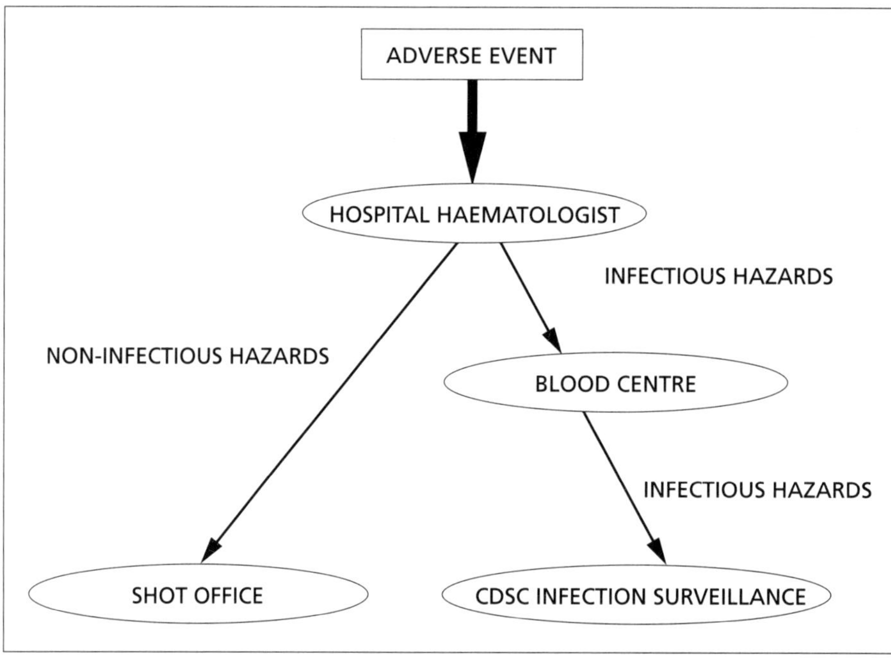

Fig. 1: Mechanism of SHOT reporting. (CDSC – Communicable Disease Surveillance Centre).

379/413 (92 %) of eligible hospitals participated in 2001/02. 199 hospitals submitted reports of incidents, and 188 indicated they had no adverse incidents by submitting a 'nil to report' form. There has been an increase every year in the number of reports, from 169 in 1996/97 to 315 in 2001/02. This may be due to better reporting or a real increase in the number of incidents; the latter is thought to be less likely, but cannot be excluded.

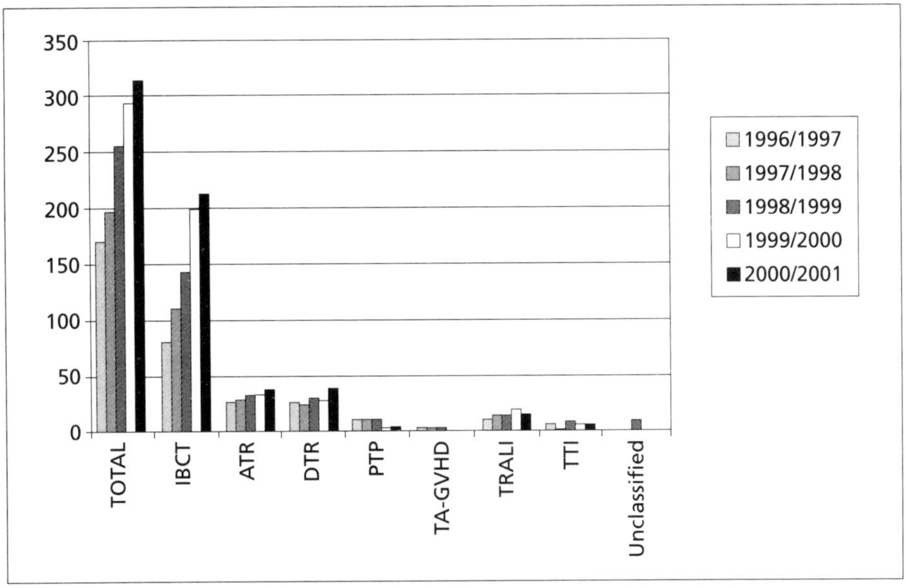

Fig. 2: Type and number of adverse events 1996/7 to 2000/01.
(IBCT – Incorrect blood component transfused; ATR – acute transfusion reaction; DHTR – delayed transfusion reaction; PTP – post-transfusion purpura; TA-GVHD – transfusion-associated graft-versus-host-disease; TRALI – transfusion-related acute lung injury; TTI – transfusion transmitted infection)

Types and frequency of adverse events

The types and frequency of adverse events are shown in Figure 2. It is striking that the most frequent event is incorrect blood transfused (IBCT). Immune complications of transfusion are all represented to varying degree, but episodes of transfusion-transmitted infection are infrequent.

The increase in reports over the five years of the scheme is due to an increase in incidents of IBCT. The number of reports of post-transfusion purpura (PTP) and transfusion-associated graft-versus-host disease (TA-GvHD) have lessened, possibly associated with the introduction of universal leucocyte-reduction of blood components in the U.K. in 1999. The incidence of the other immune events and transfusion-transmitted infection have stayed fairly constant.

Consequences of adverse events

Data on the outcome of the adverse events are shown in Figure 3. In over 70 % of cases, there was minor or no morbidity. However, 14 % of incidents were associated with major morbidity e.g. admission to an intensive care unit, renal dysfunction, or confirmed infection. The death of the patient was definitely attributed to transfusion in 37 cases (3 %), and was possibly associated with transfusion in a further 32 cases (2 %). The most frequent cause of death was TA-GvHD (13 cases). The most frequent cause of death or major morbidity was IBCT (71 cases) followed by TRALI (67 cases).

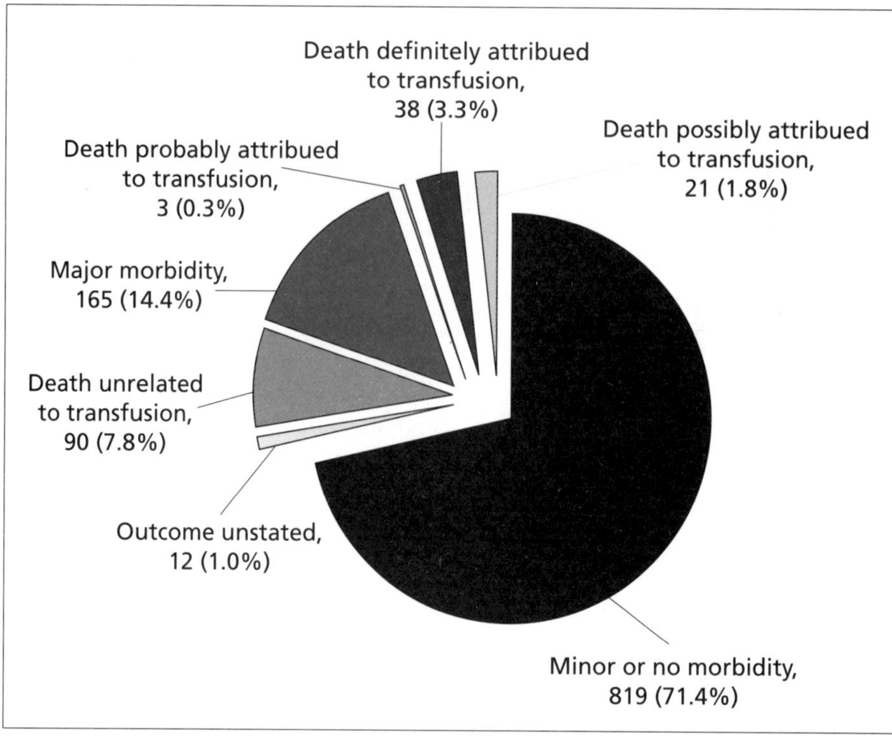

Fig. 3: Mortality and morbidity associated with adverse transfusion events (total number – 1148) reported to SHOT between 1996/97 and 2000/01.

Incorrect Blood Component Transfused (IBCT)

The SHOT scheme defines IBCT as an episode where a patient was transfused with blood which did not meet the appropriate requirements or was intended for another patient. Out of the 699 incidents reported between 1996/97 and 2000/01, there were 161 ABO incompatible transfusions (resulting in nine deaths and 37 cases of major morbidity), 73 RhD incompatible transfusions, and 37 cases involving other red cell incompatibilities. 195 wrong transfusions were by chance ABO and RhD compatible. There were 122 transfusions where special requirements such as for CMV-seronegative or gamma-irradiated blood were not met.

The causes of IBCT are shown in Figure 4. Analysis of the distribution of errors causing IBCT shows that they occur throughout the transfusion process, as has been found in other haemovigilance schemes. The most frequent site of error was found to be at the time of collection and/or administration of blood (55 %), followed by errors in the laboratory (28 %), and errors at the time of request, sampling or prescription of blood (13 %). The SHOT data have clearly demonstrated that multiple errors often contribute to IBCT; in 2001/02, 54 % of IBCT cases involved multiple errors. IBCT was found to occur in all sites where blood is used, with both elective and emergency transfusion, and to involve many types and grades of staff.

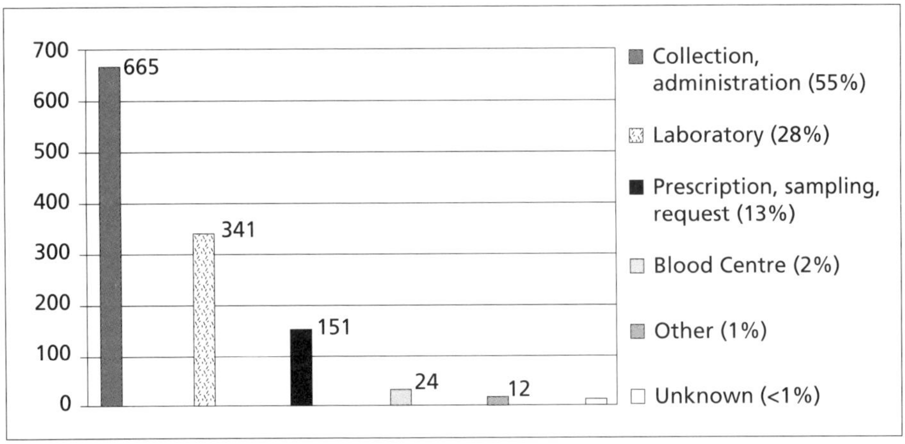

Fig. 4: Distribution of errors in incorrect blood component transfused (IBCT) incidents (total number – 699) reported to SHOT between 1996/97 and 2000/01.

IBCT incidents in 2001/02 included:-

- major intravascular haemolysis due to ABO incompatibility in two patients due to the samples for pre-transfusion testing being collected from the wrong patients.
- an increase in the proportion of IBCT caused by errors in the laboratory. The errors involved all aspects of blood banking. The most frequent error was the selection and issue of inappropriate components e.g. incorrect units for patients with known antibodies. About one third of the laboratory errors occurred out of normal working hours, with half of these involving staff who did not work regularly in the blood bank.
- many errors in collection of blood, as highlighted in the first SHOT report [3], and at the time of administration e.g. failing to detect errors earlier in the process, and failure of bedside checking that the unit is the right one for the patient. Some of these errors involved patients without identification wrist-bands, carrying out pre-transfusion identification checks remote from the bedside, and/or allowing the checking process to be disrupted by other demands.
- 32 cases of failure to request gamma-irradiated or CMV-seronegative blood components where they were indicated; fortunately, there were no complications from any of these episodes.

Transfusion-Transmitted Infection

SHOT has received 35 incidents of transfusion-transmitted infection and 38 infected recipients reported in five years. As with all the categories, it is difficult to be certain of the level of under-reporting.

The most frequent problem was bacterial infection (21/35 of the reports); it was associated with platelet transfusion in 17 cases. In many cases, skin contaminants from the donor's arm were confirmed to be the source of the contamination.

7/8 of the HBV incidents were associated with donors with acute HBV infection, and one was transmitted by a donor with chronic infection.

Near-Miss Events

SHOT has also introduced near-miss reporting. A 'near-miss' event is defined as one which, if undetected, would result in the determination of the wrong blood group for the patient, or in the issue, collection or administration of the wrong or inappropriate blood component, but which was recognised before the transfusion took place. Analysis of these errors may highlight weak points in the transfusion process. Unfortunately, near-miss reporting is taking time to become established in the SHOT scheme, and only 29 % of hospitals provided reports in 2000/01.

Sampling errors have been the most frequently reported near-miss event, usually involving the finding that the patient has a different blood group from the historical record ('wrong blood in tube').

Recommendations for Transfusion Safety

The main general recommendations from SHOT are as follows:

(i) participation in SHOT by all hospitals where blood is transfused;

(ii) encouragement of error reporting without fear of disciplinary action;

(iii) implemention of training of all staff involved in blood transfusion, and employment of sufficient numbers of nurses, laboratory staff, and doctors to enable safe and effective transfusion practice;

(iv) examination of transfusion procedures for flaws which can be corrected;

(v) support for the appropriate use of blood, although SHOT is not directly involved in this aspect of transfusion;

(vi) the establishment of an overarching framework to assess and prioritise blood safety initiatives.

SHOT has also made a number of specific recommendations, including that:-

(i) every patient should have their unique identification on a wristband;

(ii) every hospital must have a policy for the transfusion process, including bedside checking and monitoring of patients receiving transfusions;

(iii) research should be carried out into information technology solutions for safer transfusion, and into new strategies for reducing bacterial contamination and transfusion-related acute lung injury (TRALI).

Overall Progress

The SHOT scheme has accumulated substantial data on adverse transfusion incidents over a five-year period, and has made many recommendations to improve the safety of transfusion (see previous section). The rate of participation in the SHOT scheme by hospitals has steadily risen, possibly due to heightened awareness of the scheme and its importance, greater confidence in its anonymity, and pressure to participate from the Department of Health through the issue of 'Health Service Circulars' on Better Blood Transfusion to hospitals [4,5].

A number of other national haemovigilance systems has now been established worldwide [1,6,7]. Problem areas for haemovigilance schemes such as SHOT include under-reporting, possibly due to a lack of recognition of adverse events because of poor staff knowledge or fear of disciplinary action by staff if they were to report human errors. Other weaknesses of haemovigilance include failure to detect subtle adverse effects of transfusion such as immunosuppression, lack of data collection of the adverse effects of alternatives to transfusion such as the use of recombinant erythropoietin or cell salvage procedures, and a means of documentation of under-transfusion [6,7].

It would not be correct to claim that transfusion is safer in the U.K. since the inception of the SHOT scheme. However, SHOT has contributed to raising the profile of blood transfusion in the U.K., and its data provide the basis for further efforts and research into the prevention of adverse events related to transfusion.

Implementation of the Lessons Learnt from Haemovigilance

One of the major potential benefits of haemovigilance is the provision of data on which decisions about priorities for blood safety can be made. However, the process of realigning efforts to improve transfusion safety with the observed risks is no simple matter [8]. A process for decision-making might include:

(i) the development of options to deal with each major risk, or agreeing that one or more risk cannot be solved;

(ii) deciding which options are doable and affordable;

(iii) the development of an action plan.

The SHOT scheme has no mechanism for implementing its recommendations, and is reliant on other organisations to do so [7]. Furthermore, a consistent recommendation from the reports of the SHOT scheme has been the need to develop an over-arching framework for assessing transfusion hazards and prioritising blood safety initiatives. While this is still not in place in the U.K., there have been discussions about a broader remit for the U.K.'s Department of Health's Advisory Committee for the Micobiological Safety of Blood and Tissues. In the meantime, some parallel initiatives have supported the work of the SHOT scheme, including the development of national guidelines for transfusion practice by the British Committee for Standards in Haematology, for example on the administration of blood [9].

Better Blood Transfusion is an initiative led by the U.K.'s Chief Medical Officers to improve the safety and effectiveness of transfusion practice. Its output has been a number of recommended actions to hospital Chief Executives, including the establishment of Hospital Transfusion Committees (HTCs) and Hospital Transfusion Teams (HTTs). HTTs meet more regularly than HTCs, and have the task of implementing the agreed actions recommended by the HTC; they are led by a senior doctor interested in transfusion medicine (not necessarily a haematologist) and include a Transfusion Nurse, senior laboratory staff and specialists who work in clinical areas with large or high risk blood usage. The main work of these groups is directed to:

(i) the provision of training, including the development of self-learning packages, and competency testing;

(ii) the development and implementation of local policies for safe and appropriate transfusion based on national guidelines;

(iii) the provision of better information for patients.

The Chief Medical Officer's National Blood Transfusion Committee (NBTC) was established in England in 2001 (for details, see http://www.dh.gov.uk/PolicyAndGuidance/HealthAndSocialCareTopics/BloodSafety/BloodSafetyGeneralInformation/BloodSafetyGeneralArticle/fs/en). It provides a potentially powerful framework through Regional Transfusion Committees for improving transfusion practice by supporting the work of the HTCs. It oversees the national Better Blood Transfusion initiative, and acts as the Steering Group for an initiative for national comparative audit of clinical transfusion practice based on an earlier pilot scheme [10]. The NBTC reviews the findings of the SHOT scheme, and supports its recommendations. One of its main roles is to provide educational material for hospitals and patients; for example it has recently developed a national patient information leaflet (available on http://www.dh.gov.uk/PolicyAndGuidance/HealthAndSocialCareTopics/BloodSafety/BloodSafetyGeneralInformation/fs/en).

The SHOT scheme has welcomed another complementary initiative, the National Patient Safety Agency (NPSA) which was established in 2001 with a broad remit to improve the safety and quality of healthcare through reporting, analysing and learning from adverse incidents and 'near misses'. The SHOT scheme is working closely with the NPSA to avoid duplication of reporting, and ensure that lessons can be learnt from experience in other clinical areas and common solutions developed. An example of this is the use of barcode technology for patient identification and for the confirmation that the right blood will be transfused [11]. A barcode patient identification system was recently found to simplify the clinical transfusion process and improve practice [12]. These results provide support for further work on the development of such systems for transfusion, and for other hospital procedures requiring patient identification such as drug administration.

Acknowledgements

The author acknowledges that this review has been based on the data and recommendations from the reports of the SHOT scheme (available on www.shotuk.org).

References

1 Faber JC: Haemovigilance around the world. Vox Sang 2002; 83 (Suppl.1): 71-76.

2 Serious Hazards of Transfusion. Annual report 2000-2001. Serious Hazards of Transfusion Scheme, Manchester, U.K., 2002, (www.shotuk.org).

3 Serious Hazards of Transfusion. Annual report 1996-1997. Serious Hazards of Transfusion Scheme, Manchester, U.K., 1998, (www.shotuk.org).

4 Department of Health: Health Services Circular (HSC 1998/224). Better Blood Transfusion, 1998, (www.doh.gov.uk/bbt2).

5 Department of Health: Health Services Circular (HSC 2002/009). Better Blood Transfusion – Appropriate Use of Blood, 2002, (www.doh.gov.uk/bbt2).

6 Andreu G, Morel P, Forestier F, et al: Haemovigilance network in France: organization and analysis of immediate transfusion incident reports from 1994 to 1998. Transfusion 2002; 42: 1356-1364.

7 Williamson LM: Transfusion hazard reporting: powerful data, but do we know how best to use it? Transfusion 2002; 42: 1249-1252.

8 Aubuchon JP, Kruskall MS: Transfusion safety: realigning efforts with risks. Transfusion 1997; 37: 1211-1216.

9 British Committee for Standards in Haematology: The administration of blood and blood components and the management of transfused patients. Transfusion Medicine 1999; 9: 227-238.

10 Murphy MF, Wilkinson J, Lowe D, Pearson M: National audit of the transfusion process. Transfusion Medicine 2001; 11: 363-370.

11 Dzik S, Corwin H, Goodnough LT et al: Patient safety and blood transfusions: new solutions. Transfusion Medicine Reviews 2003 (in press).

12 Turner C, Casbard AC, Murphy MF: Barcode technology: its role in increasing the safety of blood transfusion. Transfusion 2003 (in press).

Professor M.F. Murphy, National Blood Service, Department of Haematology, John Radcliffe Hospital, Oxford, and the University of Oxford, Oxford OX3 9BQ, U.K.
E-mail: mike.murphy@nbs.nhs.uk

Vyas GN, Williams AE (eds): Advances in Transfusion Safety.
Dev Biol (Basel). Basel, Karger, 2005, vol 120, pp 189-195.

U.S. Regulatory Efforts to Address Errors in Transfusion

R.M. Lewis

Lorettsville, VA, USA

All those involved in the blood industry, regulator, collector, prescriber or transfusionist, have as the common goal the proper administration of a life-saving product. Over the last decade we have seen tremendous efforts and concomitant improvement in removing infectious agents from the blood supply. We currently see the need to address other areas as well; a number of authors in this volume have pointed out the need to address errors in transfusion. Transfusion errors account for one of the primary causes of transfusion-associated fatality. The FDA is currently proposing regulations to address errors and other adverse events related to blood transfusion. Those regulations, proposed in March of 2003, will be described as part of the actions the FDA is taking in recognition of the importance and seriousness of errors in transfusion in the United States.

To put the risk of transfusions error in perspective, it can be compared to the rates of infectious disease.

Hepatitis C is estimated to infect about one unit per 1.2 million units of blood; HIV one in 2 million; bacterial contamination, one in 3,000 for random donor units; bacterial contamination in red cells, around one in 30,000. Errors in administration based on Dr. Jean Linden's studies in New York State, where the state collects data on all blood transfusions, ABO incompatible blood transfusions are about one in 38,000 (Table 1). ABO compatible transfusions that are otherwise in error, are one in 41,000, with a total adjusted rate to about one in 14,000 units resulting in erroneous administration, and about one in 2 million result in a fatality. This rate compares to post-mini-pool risk for HIV.

Fatalities Associated with Blood Transfusion

The FDA currently requires the reporting of all fatalities that are associated with blood transfusion. The regulations require reporting fatalities to the FDA as soon as possible, and that a written report must be submitted within seven days of the particular fatality.

Table 1 : Comparative risks of adverse events associated with blood products.

Viral contamination		
	Pre-nat	Post minipool NAT
Hepatitis C[1]	1 : 237,000	1:1,200,000
Hepatitis B[1]	1 : 77,000	
HTLV I & II[2]	1 : 641,000	
HIV	1:1,326,000	1:1,900,000
Bacterial contamination[3]		
Random donor platelets	1 : 3000 components (1 : 500/6 pack)	
Apheresis	1 : 2000 components	
Red blood cells	1:30,000	
Erroneous administration[4]		
ABO-incompatible	1:38,000	
ABO-compatible	1:41,000	
Total (adjusted)	1:14,000	
Fatality	1:1,800,000	

1 Busch M, Stramer S, Caglioti S, Strong M, Glynn SA, Wright D, Notari E, Dodd R, Kleinman S, for the NHLBI Retrovirus Epidemiology Donor Study (REDS).

2 Transfusion medicine bulletin, America's Blood Centers, December 2001.

3 Blajchman, IABs Int Symp Advance Trans Safety, 2003.

4 Linden, Transfusion, October 2000.

Table 2 : Fatalities reported to the FDA, 1998-2002.

	2002	**2001**	**2000**	**1999**	**1998**
Haemolytic transfusion reactions/ABO	14.7 %	13.2 %	14.5 %	10.9 %	12.9 %
Incompatibility					
Laboratory error	4.2 %	5.3 %	6.5 %	6.3 %	7.1 %
Floor error (ER, ICU, OR)	10.5 %	7.9 %	8.0 %	4.7 %	6.1 %
RBC antibody reactions	12.6 %	10.5 %	8.0 %	6.3 %	7.1 %
Bacterial contamination	17.9 %	10.5 %	14.5 %	18.8 %	8.2 %
Other transfusion-related causes	29.5 %	40.8 %	37.1 %	34.4 %	48.2 %
TRALI, Pulm. Edema ; GVHD, TTD, et al					
TOTAL	**95**	**76**	**62**	**64**	**85**

Based on those fatality reports, haemolytic transfusion reactions associated with ABO incompatibility since 1998 are in the range of 10-15 %. Because we have such confidence in ABO testing, it is usually assumed that an incompatible transfusion is the result of error either in the laboratory or at the site of transfusion. The data have been collected for about 20 years and the rate of fatality has dropped over that time.

The ABO incompatible transfusions do not include all errors related to mistransfusion. In evaluating the type of errors leading to fatality, in 2002, approximately 1/3 were due to laboratory error and 2/3 were due to error at the site of transfusion. In comparing those fatality rates with other transfusion-related causes, this is roughly equivalent to death from bacterial contamination of the blood product. The next highest category of analysis includes TRALI, pulmonary oedema, GVHD, and transfusion-transmitted diseases.

Biological Product Deviation Reporting

The FDA collects data on biological product deviation reports (BPDRs). This type of reporting was previously referred to as "errors and accidents," but the regulation and title were changed. This change in title has been made to reflect the broader nature of the incidents that are reported. Not only are mistakes reported but unexpected occurrences over which a manufacturer may have no control are also required to be reported. While the nature of the reports was broader, the reports, which had been required for any part of manufacturing, were limited to products that have been released for distribution. Currently, the FDA requires that all licensed manufacturers of biological products, including blood, report within 45 days if there is some type of deviation from current good manufacturing practices, applicable regulations, or established standards, and an unexpected or unforeseeable event, any of which may affect the safety, purity and potency of the product.

The biological product deviation reports provide some insight as to what types of manufacturing errors are resulting in mis-transfusions.

Table 3 : Biological product reporting.

	Licensed		**Unlicensed**		**Trans. serv.**	
Type of BPD						
QC and distribution	2164	54.30 %	1064	40.00 %	517	39.60 %
Labelling	948	23.80 %	986	37.10 %	412	31.60 %
Routine testing	259	6.50 %	407	15.30 %	363	27.80 %
Component prep.	266	6.70 %	146	5.50 %	12	0.90 %
Blood collection	160	4.00 %	31	1.20 %		
Miscellaneous	137	3.40 %	2	0.10 %		
Viral testing	48	1.20 %	23	0.90 %		
TOTAL	**3928**		**2659**		**1304**	
Donor suitablility	**17870**		**2483**			

The largest category of BPDRs concerns donor suitability and post-donation information. Although some errors in the donor interview process might account for donor suitability errors, it is much less likely. I have taken donor suitability out of these calculations. In the actual manufacturing process, about 50 percent of errors reported are related to quality control and distribution and labelling errors (24 percent).

ADVERSE REACTION REPORTING

For adverse reactions that are related to blood transfusion, the FDA requires establishments to investigate the adverse reaction and to prepare and maintain a written report of the investigation, including their follow-up and conclusions; such a report, if it is a transfusion facility, has to be sent to the collecting facility (21 CFR 606.170). These reports are not sent to the FDA at a particular centralized reporting system. The requirement is limited to the investigation, follow-up action, and maintenance of the records. They are made available for the FDA inspections force.

However, FDA has proposed new regulations that address safety reporting of adverse events that may be related to blood donation or transfusion (SADR) (Safety Reporting Requirements for Human Drug and Biological Products;

Proposed Rule; Federal Register: 68 (50), 12405-12497).

In addition to the fatalities reports, described above, if the proposed rule is finalized, blood establishments would be required to report some of the most serious adverse events.

The proposed regulation would not affect the reporting of fatalities. That system would continue as it is currently structured. As such, a fatal reaction would be reported in a written report within seven calendar days of the fatality, as well as notifying us, usually by telephone, fax, or internet, as soon as possible.

As part of the proposal of the SADR for serious adverse reactions related to transfusion that do not result in a fatality, the FDA has provided a discussion of our intent in the preamble of the regulation. In addition, a number of different examples of possible effects have been listed. Four sets of examples are provided: those that might be reported, considered serious, for donation events, and those that might be reported for transfusion events. Likewise, examples were provided that might not be reported for donation or transfusion events.

Table 4a: Serious adverse reactions related to blood collection.

- Vasovagal reactions with syncope (hypotension and bradycardia) requiring medical intervention;
- Citrate reactions requiring significant medical intervention;
- Anaphylaxis or any major allergic reactions;
- Seizure of any type or duration;
- Cerebrovascular accidents;
- Cardiac arrhythmia, angina of any duration, myocardial infarction, or cardiac arrest;
- Clinically significant hypotension;
- Bronchospasm, respiratory insufficiency;
- Arterial puncture, air embolus;
- Phlebotomy-related nerve damage; and,
- Thrombophlebitis, phlebitis, or any procedure-related infection.

Table 4b: Serious adverse reactions not related to blood collection.

- Self-limited vasovagal reactions (haemodynamically stable);
- Self-limited citrate reactions;
- Localized haematoma, uncomplicated; and,
- Localized skin irritation, uncomplicated.

Table 4c: Serious adverse reactions related to blood transfusion.

- Any complication from the use of an unsuitable unit, including infusion of haemolysed blood;
- Any complication from improper blood administration, including failure to use a standard blood filter (e.g., air embolism);
- Induced haemolysis, acute or delayed;
- Transmitted infections, including bacterial infections;
- Associated graft versus host disease;
- Related hypersensitivity with respiratory insufficiency and/or hypotension (e.g., anaphylaxis);
- Transfusion-related acute lung injury (TRALI);
- Induced allo-immunization which prevents effective transfusion therapy (e.g., post-transfusion purpura);
- Induced congestive heart failure; and
- Induced cardiac arrhythmias, including those resulting from metabolic imbalance.

Table 4d: Serious adverse reactions not related to blood transfusion.

- Febrile non-haemolytic transfusion reactions;
- Related hypersensitivity without respiratory insufficiency nor hypotension;
- Induced allo-immunization which does not prevent effective transfusion therapy;
- Infections not clinically significant to the recipient, such as cytomegalovirus (CMV) infection in an immunocompetent adult;
- Induced haemochromatosis.

A number of these examples include the phrase, "requiring medical intervention." FDA has received numerous comments about this phrase suggesting that if the rule becomes final, the phrase should be better and more clearly defined. For instance, it is important in distinguishing between a common blood donation phenomenon of vaso-vagal reaction and a more serious loss of consciousness that requires a physician or emergency medical personnel to be called.

All serious adverse drug reactions, except fatalities, would be reported to the FDA within 45 calendar days. This period was chosen to coincide with the reporting for biological product deviations. It was noted that some events may fit the requirements for biological product deviation and serious adverse events. The 45 calendar day requirement would thus allow reporting facilities to investigate and draw conclusions in the same period and report at the same time.

"Bar Code" Regulation

Previous presentations, in this volume, in particular from Dr. Gerald Sandler, Dr. Harold Kaplan and Dr. Michael Murphy have referred to bar coding and how important it could be for the correct administration of blood products. In recognition of medical errors in general, Secretary of the Department of Health and Human Services, Tommy Thompson, has recognized the importance of mis-administrations for all drugs, biologicals and blood products, and has encouraged the development of the proposal for requiring drugs and biologicals to be labelled with bar code information and for blood products to be labelled with machine-readable code. This proposal, **Bar Code Label Requirements for Human Drug Products and Blood** (Federal Register: 68 (50), 12499-12534, 2003) was published at the same time as the adverse reaction reporting regulation and public comments were requested by June 12, 2003, but FDA accepts comments at any time.

Who would have to use bar codes? The FDA recognized that our authority does not extend to the hospital situation and it does not regulate medical care. However, the FDA does have authority to regulate manufacturers, re-packers, re-labellers and private label distributors for drugs and biologicals. It is these entities that will be required to implement the labelling as described in this particular regulation. The current situation in medical care regarding electronic labelling has been described as like the "chicken or the egg."

Previously, health care facilities would not implement systems to use technology for drug administration because they were not available on the particular labels of the purchased drugs. On the other hand, drug manufacturers did not put technology into their labelling because it was not demanded by the hospitals. So, in recognition of this circular set of circumstances, and the need to address errors in drug administration, the FDA has taken the first step to require that such labelling be implemented over a number of years for drugs, biologicals and blood.

For drugs and biologicals, the regulation would require a national drug code (NDC) number to be encoded on the label. The number would be issued at random by the FDA to current manufacturers or new manufacturers after submission of an application. The proposal would require that the particular bar code would be in the UCC/EAN symbology.

In recognition of errors in transfusion and serious injuries that can result from transfusion errors, as discussed above, the most common error outside blood banks is administering properly labelled blood to a patient other than the one for whom it was intended, blood products will be required to bear a machine-readable label. FDA anticipates that such action will also address the less common mislabelling of samples for patient typing and cross-matching, as well as issue of the wrong unit or testing errors.

At least two bar code technologies are available and in use in transfusion services and blood banks in the United States: Codabar and ISBT 128. The FDA has recognized the ISBT 128, developed by The International Council for Commonality in Blood Banking Automation, Inc., as acceptable, except where there are inconsistencies in the regulation. The FDA notes in guidance that there are two inconsistencies and, in its published Guidance, describes how they can be addressed (**Recognition and Use of a Standard for the Uniform Labeling of Blood and Blood Components**). The symbology for ISBT 128 is similar to, but not identical with, Code 128, which fits into the UCC symbology. Despite the international conventions and this particular guidance document, the use of ISBT 128 has not been universally implemented.

Other components of this proposal would be that all blood establishments would be subject to the machine-readable information requirement, and that blood and blood components intended for transfusion would have machine-readable information required on their particular label. The form of the code would need to be accepted by the Director, Center for Biologics Evaluation and Research.

The following information would be required to be encoded: (i) a unique facility identifier; (ii) a lot number, relating to the donor; (iii) a product code; and (iv) the donor's ABO blood group and Rh type. The products subject to this regulation would be “blood” or “blood components,” and those blood or blood components that are to be transfused to a patient, or products from which blood or blood components can be removed and transfused to a patient.

In summary, the FDA centrally collects minimal data on errors related to transfusion, but in recognition of the seriousness of this particular circumstance, it has proposed initiatives to collect data on adverse events related to blood transfusion, as well as to require that machine-readable information be placed on the labels of blood and blood components, in anticipation that health care facilities will use the labels and implement systems to protect patients from errors. It should be noted that at the time of preparation of this information the bar code and rule and the SADR rule were proposed. It is anticipated that within the next few months, the bar code regulation will be made final. In its final form, some of the principles described here might have been amended to take into consideration public comments.

I would like to acknowledge the efforts of Les Holness, Elizabeth Callaghan, Lois Simmons, Sharon O'Callaghan, and John Lee who contributed to gathering the data and information.

Dr. R.M. Lewis, 39275 Snow Lane, Lorettsville, VA 20180, USA.
E-mail: rlewis@accessbio.com

Editorial note: At the time of this presentation, the bar code regulation was still under development at the FDA. It has since become a final rule (see Federal Register 69FR9120, published 02/26/04) and the proposed provisions discussed in this chapter are now required. The reporting of adverse reactions has not become a final rule and may still be under consideration at FDA.

Vyas GN, Williams AE (eds): Advances in Transfusion Safety.
Dev Biol (Basel). Basel, Karger, 2005, vol 120, pp 197-198.

Ordering Blood for the Wrong Patient: Getting Inside the Minds of Ordering Physicians

M.L. Foss, S.B. Moore

Division of Transfusion Medicine, Mayo Clinic Rochester, MN, USA

Background

Our blood transfusion request forms contained both machine-imprinted patient identification plus a physician's handwritten version of the same identification facts. The purpose of the handwritten requirement was to force the ordering physician to consider (a second time) just who was the intended recipient, especially in a setting where the physician might be writing multiple orders (including blood orders) for many different patients. The imprinting alone of the patient's identity can be performed by others (nurses, unit clerks, etc.) who may misinterpret the physician's real intention. The retention of the imprinted identification helped ensure legibility and the detection of a discrepancy between handwritten and imprinted data. Such detection has prevented blood transfusion to unintended recipients. Most systems for the prevention of transfusion administration errors focus on ensuring that the blood ordered for patient A is given only to patient A. We realized that if the ordering physician misidentifies the **intended recipient**, then the process of blood sampling, crossmatching, and blood administration will proceed unchecked and compatible blood will be given to patient A when the intended recipient was patient B.

Methods and Results

In early 1997, at the request of clinicians, the transfusion order form was modified to eliminate the requirement for handwritten patient information. The number of blood orders for the wrong patient immediately began to increase. The figure indicates the changes in orders for the wrong patients.

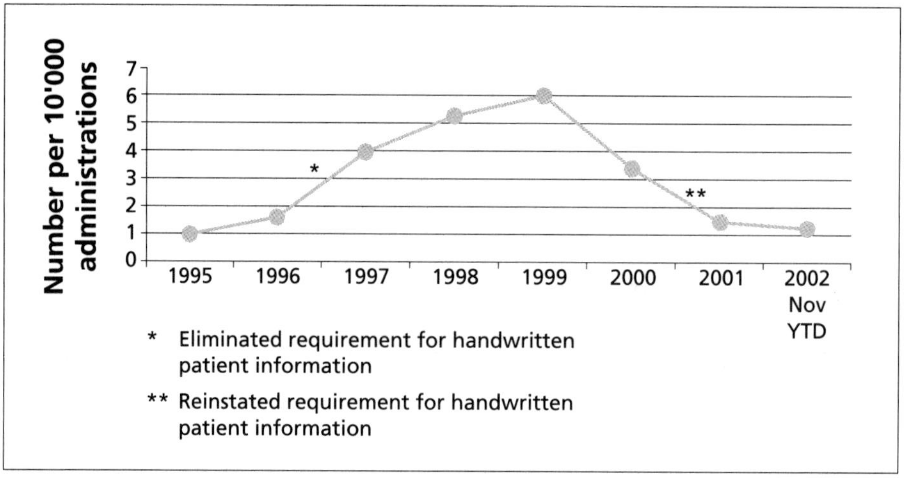

Fig. 1: Blood orders for the wrong patient.

In 1999, there were a total of 47 blood orders for the wrong patient. Of those, 33 were discovered before the blood was released from the laboratory; 11 were discovered at the bedside before transfusion; and three actually resulted in unnecessary transfusion.

The temporal relationship between the removal of handwritten information and the dramatic increase in the number of orders for the wrong patient led us, in mid-2000, to reinstate the requirement for handwritten patient information on the transfusion order form. Almost immediately the error rate went down to former low levels.

Conclusion

When the requirement for the second patient identifier (both handwritten and machine imprinted) on the blood order form was lifted, the rate at which blood was ordered for the wrong patient increased markedly. When the requirement was reinstated, the error rate went down to former levels and has remained at those levels. These data suggest that providing busy ordering physicians with a redundant "second thought" process does prevent the opportunity for beginning the process of ordering blood for an unintended recipient.

Dr. M.L. Foss, Division of Transfusion Medicine, Mayo Clinic Rochester, 200 First Street SW, Hilton 253, Rochester, MN 55905-0002, USA.
E-mail: foss.mary@mayo.edu

Vyas GN, Williams AE (eds): Advances in Transfusion Safety.
Dev Biol (Basel). Basel, Karger, 2005, vol 120, p 199.

SESSION XIV

Evidence-Based Transfusion Practice

Moderator: *H.G. Klein*

Vyas GN, Williams AE (eds): Advances in Transfusion Safety.
Dev Biol (Basel). Basel, Karger, 2005, vol 120, p 201.

RBC Transfusion Triggers: The Evidence

J.L. Carson

Division of General Internal Medicine, UMDNJ-Robert Wood Johnson Medical School, New Brunswick, NJ, USA

The indications for red cell transfusion are very controversial. Most modern guidelines conclude that transfusion therapy should be individualized, and consider the patients symptoms rather than focusing on a specific haemoglobin level. Recent trends have been to use lower thresholds for allogeneic red cell transfusions because of fears of HIV, hepatitis, and vCJD. However, the safety of allogeneic red cell transfusion has improved greatly during the past 20 years in countries with a well-regulated blood supply

The risk associated with anaemia can be estimated by examining the outcome in surgical patients who decline blood for religious reasons. We have performed a retrospective cohort study included 1,958 adult consecutive surgical patients who refused transfusion for religious reasons. In patients with underlying cardiovascular disease, we found that the risk of death was much higher than in patients without underlying cardiovascular disease as the haemoglobin level fell below 10 g/dl. Patients with perioperative haemoglobin levels below 5-6 g/dL had very high rates of mortality and morbidity.

A systematic review of the literature identified only 16 studies, which were controlled; 11 were randomized controlled trials, and five were observational studies. Only one clinical trial (Hebert et al, N Engl J Med, 1999) in ICU patients was sufficiently viable to examine clinical outcomes. This study suggested that a restrictive transfusion threshold of 7 g/dl did not adversely affect the outcome compared to a liberal transfusion threshold. All other studies were much too small. Only one study examined symptomatic transfusion.

Given the uncertain general nature of the data across different clinical settings, the limited data from patients with underlying cardiovascular disease, and the absence of data on functional recovery, additional randomized clinical trials are needed. For the present, we recommend the use of a restrictive transfusion trigger except in patients with cardiovascular disease for which higher threshold should be considered.

Dr. J.L. Carson, Division of General Internal Medicine, UMDNJ-Robert Wood Johnson Medical School, 125 Paterson St., Suite 5100, New Brunswick, NJ 08903-0019, USA
E-mail: Carson@umdnj.edu

Vyas GN, Williams AE (eds): Advances in Transfusion Safety.
Dev Biol (Basel). Basel, Karger, 2005, vol 120, pp 203-213.

The Evidence Base for Blood Donor Selection Criteria

V. James

National Blood Service, Sheffield, United Kingdom

Key words: Donor selection, evidence based guidelines

This paper will cover the following issues:

(i) The relevance of donor selection criteria for blood safety and availability. The new balance between fall in donors and rise of bloodless medicine.

(ii) Evidence Based Medicine: does this concept apply to donor selection criteria?

(iii) How are donor selection guidelines developed? (Experience from United Kingdom and Council of Europe) How should they be developed?

(iv) Blood donor deferral in England

(v) The five distinct categories of deferral criteria.

Detailed consideration of three common deferral criteria guidance: Comparison of guidelines from: AABB Uniform Donor Questionnaire, New York Blood Center, ASBP, United Kingdom, Council of Europe.

Finally collaboration is suggested which may provide the missing evidence base for some donor selection criteria.

The Relevance of Blood Donor Selection Criteria to Blood Safety and Availability

Maintaining the balance between donor blood safety and availability has preoccupied the blood services throughout the world. More recently, however, blood services are also becoming involved with the appropriate use of the blood and components they produce. The whole discipline of transfusion medicine has evolved into a clinically orientated discipline, concerned with the appropriate use of blood products. This is clearly discussed by Goodnough [1].

Interestingly the fall in donor numbers coincides with the rise in bloodless surgery and bloodless medicine and a new balance is to be achieved. A greater understanding of alternatives to allogeneic blood transfusion among traditional transfusionists is called for. Recent issues of Transfusion have carried numerous papers on approaches to alternative solutions.

In England the National Blood Service has developed a multidisciplinary approach to encouraging the use of a wide portfolio of alternatives to allogeneic blood. This move was precipitated by the concerns over expected falls in donors due to worries about vCJD but it soon became clear that this approach would inevitably lead to better blood transfusion practice and also meet patient expectations of avoidance of allogeneic transfusion. The Department of Health produced an excellent Health Service Circular: Better Blood Transfusion Appropriate Use of Blood (Ref. HSC 2002/009) which actually sets a programme of action for health service managers with a timetable for expected achievements.

To understand fully the new balance between availability of donor blood and safety we first need to understand demand. It remains very difficult, if not impossible, to assess the real need for allogeneic blood products. Edward L. Wallace, in the recent editorial in Transfusion "Monitoring the Nation's blood supply", ref. [2] states: "Evaluation for the success of these (monitoring) efforts depends on how the terms of adequacy and shortage are measured". A multiplicity of events can be used to define an actual shortage or threat of shortage. At the moment we simply do not know how much donor blood is actually required; most Services estimate a comfortable stock which ensures a minimal failure to supply. In England this is currently set at four days' stock, but is generally exceeded. To achieve such stock levels needs donors and throughout the world donors are increasingly difficult to attract and retain.

Simon [3] suggests two main reasons for this for the U.S., equally applicable in U.K.: increased restrictions for blood donors and length and burden of the donor questionnaire. He points out that "the full impact of exclusion on numbers of donors has never been fully investigated". "Once restrictions became a part of the blood donor questionnaire it was extremely difficult to eliminate them if epidemiological evidence indicated that they are of no use".

He suggests that it is "necessary to reopen the gates of donation". Basing donor selection criteria on available evidence can help to open these gates. In the U.K. we are currently examining the evidence base for donor selection criteria to avoid loss of donations without jeopardising the safety of either the donor or the recipient.

Evidence Based Medicine: Does this Concept Apply to Donor Selection Criteria?

Clinical transfusion is already moving towards solid evidence-based practice, witness the numerous guidelines and the fall in transfusion trigger from 12g/dl to 7-8 g/dl. However the guidelines for donor selection lag far behind in using evidence based criteria.

What is evidence based medicine?

The criteria for assessing and grading evidence were first proposed by the U.S. Institute of Medicine in 1990 [4].

As always happens with useful instruments, the users tinker and modify, so now many different classifications are in use but all share the principles of stating the level of evidence on which the recommendations are based. Levels of evidence are generally also taken from the original work but often sub-classifications are used.

The classification adopted by the BCSH (British Committee for Standards in Haematology) is the following:

Statements of evidence

Grade	Level	Statement
A	Ia	Evidence obtained from meta-analysis of randomised controlled trials.
	Ib	Evidence obtained from at least one randomised controlled trial.
B	IIa	Evidence obtained from at least one well-designed controlled study without randomisation.
	IIb	Evidence obtained from at least one other type of well-designated quasi-experimental study.
C	III	Evidence obtained from well-designed non-experimental descriptive studies, such as comparative studies, correlation studies and case studies.
	IV	Evidence obtained from expert committee reports or opinions and/or clinical experiences of respected authorities.

A, B and C refer to grades of recommendation.

Evidence level IV, the lowest level, brings in the experts.

Who are the Experts? Where is the expertise?

A symposium with this title was held in 2002 [5], the conclusion being that "expertise is attained on a base of knowledge, guided by experience". This definition allows patients as well as clinicians to be experts. It is also pointed out that expertise is divisive because it is founded on exclusivity; by definition the attributes that make someone an expert are not shared by others.

What is the relationship between guidelines and evidence base?

Guidelines are defined as: "systematically developed statements to assist practitioners and patients in decisions about appropriate health care for specific clinical circumstances. Their purpose is to "make explicit recommendations with a definite intent to influence what clinicians do". "The link between a set of guidelines and the scientific evidence must be explicit and scientific and clinical evidence should take precedence over expert judgement".

Guidelines now abound, and possibly the very profusion of these leads to uncertainty so that clinical compliance with guidelines remains a problem area.

- In England, U.K.: NICE www.nice.org (National Institute of Clinical Excellence)
- In Scotland U.K.: SIGN www.sign.ac.uk (Scottish Intercollegiate Guideline Network)

- In Europe: AGREE www.agreecollaboration.org (Appraisal of Guidelines for Research and Evaluation), a multinational collaboration. AGREE have provided a framework for assessing the quality of clinical practice guidelines.
- In the U.S.: National Guideline Clearinghouse www.guideline.gov

Evidence-based medicine has its critics, the most humorous of which are Clinicians for the Restoration of Autonomous Practice. More serious criticism questions the validity of the evidence and the lack of availability of the data on which the evidence is assessed. A common-sense approach is taken by Haynes. "Evidence does not make decisions, people do" [6] states: clinicians should pay due respect, no more, to current best evidence in making decisions.

Donor selection guidelines should take account of the evidence base; even if the levels of available evidence cannot reach levels I and II, we can still do better than remain at evidence level IV.

How Are Donor Selection Guidelines Developed? How Should they be Developed?

The U.K. is one Member State in the European Union (15 nations, recently expanded to 25 in May 2004). The U.K. also comprises four separate countries. In 1997 there was devolution of governments for England, Wales, Scotland, Northern Ireland. This led to the establishment of four blood/blood transfusion services, one in each country; they are administratively different and lines of accountability lead to different management boards. Between them - these four Services collect all the blood in the U.K. - there are no other organisations involved. However, since 1989 we have had one structured organisation with responsibility for producing and updating the guidelines for the four Services: The Professional Advisory Committee joint with the National Institute for Biological Standards and Control (JPAC). The four Services therefore, although different, abide by the same guidelines. Strictly, they do not have to do so until the EU Directive 2002/98/EC setting standards of quality and safety for the collection, testing, processing, storage and distribution of human blood and blood components, comes into force in 2005.

JPAC has a family of Standing Advisory Committees and Working Parties. More than 100 professionals from the four Services, NIBSC, hospitals and universities in the U.K. are involved. We still need lay stakeholder participation. The donor selection guidelines are developed by one of these Standing Advisory Committees whose role is to monitor developments world-wide, discuss their relevance to the U.K., reach conclusions and advise the four Services. The Services are responsible for any implementation and they are at liberty not to implement but are well advised to justify their non-compliance. All the U.K. guidelines can be found on www.transfusionguidelines.org.uk

Most of the donor selection guidelines are based on time-honoured "custom and practice," and only now are we scrutinising the evidence base for these.

Over the years the U.K. has worked very closely with the Council of Europe (an organisation distinct from and not to be confused with the European Union, with 45 member states). The CoE donor selection guidelines and those in the U.K. are very similar, if not identical. The EU is currently accepting the work of the CoE in this area [7], but the detailed technical requirements which will specify donor selection criteria are still in the consultation process. In 2005 the agreed technical requirements will become law in the Member States and it is vitally important that the donor selection criteria are based on available evidence and allow rapid modification should the evidence indicate a need to change.

How should the donor selection guidelines be developed?

It is clear that guidelines are needed for developing and assessing the guidelines themselves. The AGREE collaboration has provided a suitable framework.

Blood Donor Deferral in England

One advantage of a National Service in England is that uniform data can be collected throughout the country which can be analysed and changes made based on available data.

April 2002 - April 2003: Whole blood

Over $2^1/_2$ million donors attended to donate blood in England. 14 % of attendances did not result in a donation, approximately half due to low Hb incomplete donation/failed venepuncture, and the other half because donors were deferred.

In all, approximately 160,000 donors were deferred because they did not meet our donor selection guidelines. The highest proportion was due to some medical problem at the time of donation, having had skin piercing, or an unacceptable travel history. A common medical problem was a history of high blood pressure. Over 5,000 donors were deferred for this reason.

These are very large numbers of donors, some deferred permanently, others for short periods. There are two key questions we need to ask:

(i) are the guidelines correct?

(ii) are they correctly applied?

A national audit [8] was carried out over a two-week period in 2001 to try and answer the second question.

107,224 donors attended and 8,810 were deferred (8.2 %, higher than the national data for 2002). Of these, 2,335 (2.1 %, were first time donors and donors who had not attended for two years. The main reasons for deferral were travel, minor illness and skin piercing.

131 (5.6 % of deferrals) were deemed to be inappropriate.

131 inappropriate deferrals in a 2-week period becomes a large number in the year. This issue is being addressed through clarifying the current guidelines and training of staff.

However, the correctness of the guidelines also needs to be addressed.

(i) travel: an issue of estimated risk is difficult

(ii) minor illness: an issue of complexity of the guidelines and individual judgement and staff training;

(iii) skin piercing: deferral period should take account of the improvement in tests (HCV-NAT has enabled us to reduce this from 12 months to12 weeks).

The Five Distinct Categories of Donor Deferral Criteria

I have used this division for simplicity, while fully aware of its shortcomings.

5.1. Donors with a condition known to be transmitted by blood;

5.2. Donors at risk of acquiring a condition transmitted by blood;

5.3. Donors with a condition where transmissibility has been by unknown blood;

5.4. Donors at risk of a condition where transmissibility is by blood unknown;

Donors whose own health might be damaged by donating.

As always there are several conditions which belong to more than one category and it would be an interesting exercise to make a list of these, thus forcing us to think more clearly about exactly why we use them.

5.1. Donors with conditions known to be transmitted by blood

These are the issues most often discussed at any blood safety meeting. In general all developed transfusion services apply all of these (ex: HIV, HBV, HCV, HTLV). However rules vary for syphilis, a documented transfusion transmissible infection, where the donor eligibility rules vary; some services accepting treated donors, others deferring permanently or for various periods, either because it is still regarded as a proxy test of an unacceptable lifestyle, or to prevent embarrassment to the donor whose blood tests reveal past infection. To my knowledge a clear evidence base does not exist for either reason.

5.2. Donors who are at risk of acquiring a condition transmissible by blood

The arguments here focus on risk and, equally important, perception of risk.

The importance of communication in assessing risk, well known in the commercial field, is gaining recognition in transfusion medicine [9,10].

Numerous catch-phrases have crept into the language: "zero risk", "theoretical risk", "safe", "no evidence of risk is not evidence of risk", the "precautionary principle". Graphs and pictures putting the risk of receiving a transfusion in the context of other everyday risks have helped communication [11,12].

The European School of Transfusion Medicine held a three-day meeting in 2000 entitled "Risk perception and risk assessment in transfusion medicine", and a symposium exploring the concept of acceptable risk was held in London in 2000 [13].

However, none of these risk analysis tools has helped when we are faced as today with SARS and WNV. Travel bans are established rapidly. The problem is that acceptable risk, both by patients and the professionals, has not and possibly cannot be defined. Hence, a precautionary principle is evoked and as a consequence numerous donations are lost.

In the U.K. we have life exclusion for men who have sex with men. This has been queried and quite rightly the affected potential donors have asked for a clear explanation and justification of this stance.

A careful epidemiological study by Kate Soldan [14,15] putting figures on the risks of HIV-positive donations entering the blood supply, should these rules be relaxed, has recently been published.

The data presented in these papers have helped communicate the reasoning of the transfusion services to homosexual men and the general public in the U.K.

5.3. Donors with conditions where the transmissibility by blood is unknown or not established

Here the focus is on attempting to establish transmissibility ; for obvious reasons the work relies on historical accidental data, or animal work. The current difficulties in establishing transmissibility of vCJD by blood and components in humans lead to serious ethical issues, concerned with confidentiality.

Example for analysis:

Cancer

AABB UDHQ:	Question 43: Have you ever had any type of cancer, including leukaemia? A donor with a history of cancer must be evaluated/deemed eligible to donate: Refer to SOP.
ASBP:	localised skin cancer (basal cell carcinoma or squamous cell carcinoma,) acceptable if completely excised and healed). Carcinoma in situ of cervix: acceptable. Malignant melanoma, leukaemia, lymphoma. Hodgkin's disease: permanent deferral. All others require medical director's approval.
NYBC:	Same criteria as for ASBP. Other causes: (there is no mention of medical director's approval) Carcinoma in remission for at least five years except where noted.
U.K.:	Accept: Basal cell carcinoma skin (rodent ulcer). C. in situ cervix when treated. Permanently exclude individuals with a history of malignant disease.
CoE:	Individuals with a malignant disease or a history of such are usually permanently deferred. Physicians in charge may make exceptions to this, for example a donor may be accepted at the conclusion of successful treatment for non-invasive cervical cancer & rodent ulcer.

These rules are not based on any acceptable evidence, more on medical "gut feeling".

It would help if all transfusion services could work together and gather whatever data those centres that have accepted donors with a past history of malignancy can provide.

5.4. Donors at risk of a condition where transmissibility by blood is unknown

This is the most complex area and introduces requirements for both analysis of risk and assumptions about transmissibility.

Examples are: donors with a family history of CJD, donors with genetic predispositions to cancers, lifestyle risk in donors with predispositions to cancers.

Should we defer all smokers or some smokers?

5.5. Donors with conditions where the act of donation may cause them harm

These conditions are very numerous and have generally escaped scrutiny. Many are dogma, even more are made at donor sessions by caring and concerned staff, often based on their personal experience. They include a wide range of illnesses (asthma, epilepsy, coughs, colds, etc.) and other issues such as eating or not before donation, and exercising or pursuing hazardous hobbies after donation. Almost all such restrictions are based on custom and practice, the "what if donor has delayed faint?" or expert opinion.

They result in a vast number of lost donations and donors, offended by being rejected for reasons which appear nonsensical to them and where the only explanation offered is "it is our rule".

Just three more will be further compared: pregnancy, blood pressure, and diabetes mellitus. Chosen as prevalent and therefore resulting in the greatest number of lost donations. The guidelines are quoted verbatim to highlight the shorthand used which makes for ambiguity.

Example 1: Pregnancy

AABB UDHQ	and user guide: question 7. In the past week have you been pregnant or are you pregnant now? Eligibility: a female with a known pregnancy or who has been pregnant in the last six weeks should not donate blood. Defer according to SOP.
ASBP:	Defer during pregnancy and for six weeks after delivery or termination
NYBC:	Defer during pregnancy and for six weeks after full term delivery or miscarriage/termination after 1st Trimester (12 weeks).
CoE:	Pregnant women should not be accepted other than in exceptional circumstances and at the discretion of the physician in charge of the pregnancy. Following pregnancy, the deferral period should last as many months as the duration of the pregnancy or at least throughout the lactation period.
U.K.:	Obligatory: if pregnancy resulted in a hydatidiform mole, permanently exclude if malignant (invasive) otherwise defer until treatment and follow-up is completed. See: blood transfusion Discretionary: defer during pregnancy and then one week for every completed week of pregnancy.

Basically the U.S. accepts donors six weeks after delivery, the U.K. and CoE leave it for 40 weeks. Clearly these rules are not evidence-based.

In England there were 584,000 live births in 1999 (data from the Office of National Statistics). Even if 1 % of these mothers wished to donate, and we used the U.S. six-week deferral rule, we could have had 5,800 donations, or given that two could have been obtained in the period six to 40 weeks, over 10,000 donations. It is more likely that in this group, 10 % would willingly donate, thus increasing the donations to 100,000 or more.

What is needed for the U.K. and the Council of Europe to change the 40-week deferral rule? Evidence that donors come to no harm and their donations will not cause harm.

Where can we obtain this evidence? By asking the U.S. for information on adverse events in donors attending six weeks post delivery, and also any which indicate a higher risk to the recipient.

Collaborative work is needed. Even then differences in population customs and nutritional state will not make the data comparable; but it is better than no data.

Example 2: Blood pressure

AABB UDHQ:	Two questions might bring this to light. Q1: Are you feeling healthy and well today? If NO consult SOP. Q 44: Have you had any problems with your heart or lungs? If YES: consult SOP.
ASBP:	High Blood Pressure: donor systolic must be ≤ 180, Diastolic ≤ 100 Hypertension: accept if controlled with medication and BP at time of donation is within guidelines.
NYBC:	Hypertension: accept if blood pressure at site is within NYBC guidelines (P & D Manual). Hypotension: accept if blood pressure at site is within NYBC guidelines (P & D Manual).
CoE:	It is recommended that pulse and blood pressure be tested. It is recognised that recording the blood pressure may be subject to several variables but as a guide the systolic should not exceed 180 mm Hg and the diastolic 100mm Hg.
U.K.:	Blood pressure high: exclude permanently if on treatment even if blood pressure is normal on treatment. Exception: accept if treatment with diuretics only and only if otherwise in good health. Blood pressure low: accept if the donor is not prone to faints or dizzy spells.

This was one of the conditions for which the Standing Advisory Committee was asked to gather the evidence base as a priority because of concerns at the wording of the Council of Europe Guidelines which involved routine taking of blood pressure for all donors and the possibility that the CoE recommendations become part of a legally binding technical requirements in the EU.

Hypertension is prevalent in the U.K.; it is estimated that 20 % of the population are hypertensive, of whom 60 % are on treatment (Office of National Statistics).

The first questions asked was: why should blood pressure be considered at all as a donor selection criterion?

Answer 1: could a hypertensive or hypotensive donor come to harm by donating?

Answer 2: useful population screening and meets donor expectation

For neither of these was there any evidence. The British Hypertensive Society was consulted and the following answers were given:

"It is not necessary for BP to be measured routinely before blood donation. We are scraping the barrel for justification of an unnecessary procedure in the context of routine blood donation".

"The circumstances of measurement are such that any measurement is meaningless". Are these statements evidence-based or expert opinion? Evidence, as expected these days, is simply not available and cannot be gathered, except again by comparing practice and gathering the data. The wording of the Council of Europe guidelines was changed to remove the recommendation as a routine procedure on the basis of the expert opinions gathered from clinicians dealing directly with hypertension.

Example 3: Diabetes Mellitus

AABB UDHQ:	Question 4: have you ever taken any medication on the Medical Deferral list (beef insulin from U.K.)? Indefinite deferral
NYBC:	accept if diet controlled and/or on oral hypoglycaemics
	accept if on insulin (including insulin pump) and stable (donor must have eaten before donation)
ASBP:	Accept if on oral hypoglycaemics or insulin, if dosage controlled and stable unless bovine insulin has been used any time since 1980.
CoE:	permanently defer if requires insulin.
U.K.:	permanently exclude if on medication (accept if controlled by diet and otherwise in good health).

In England there are 1.15 million diabetics (National Office of Statistics), most of whom do not qualify as blood donors, merely because of the insulin treatment they receive.

What is required to change the CoE and hence U.K. guidelines in this respect?

Answer: evidence from countries where diabetics on insulin are accepted that neither they nor the recipients of their blood/components come to any harm.

The issue here is more complex because these patients are at greater risk of infection than pregnant women or hypertensives, so clear evidence that the donations are no more likely to transmit infection than the standard will also be needed.

In Conclusion

The examples, if followed through, will benefit the European Blood Services. Areas where U.S. selection criteria are more stringent, and hence Europe could provide data, are around travel history and a history of hepatitis. But it seems that in the U.S. many decisions are left to medical directors and a careful look at these inevitably varying decisions, gathering the data and reaching clearer evidence by comparing practice, will avoid the loss of valuable donations. We cannot experiment with donors, but the experiments are going on all the time; all we need do is formalise the experience we are gathering daily.

We also need to involve the public (of which we are part) in defining "acceptable risk", and finally we need to have the courage to change our donor selection criteria in line with the knowledge we gain.

References

1 Goodnough LT, Shander A, Brecher ME: Transfusion medicine: looking to the future. The Lancet 2003; 361: 161-169.

2 Wallace EL: Monitoring the nation's blood supply. Transfusion 2003; 43 (3): 299-301.

3 Simon TL: Where have all the donors gone? A personal reflection on the crisis in America's volunteer blood program. Transfusion 2003; 43 (2): 273-279.

4 Field MJ, Lohr KN (eds): Institute of Medicine Committee to advise the public Health Service in clinical practice guidelines: directions for a new program. Washington DC, National Academy Press.

5 Drug and Therapeutics Bulletin 2002; 40: 55-56.

6 Haynes RB, Devereaux PJ, Guyatt GH: Physicians' and patients' choices in evidence based practice. BMJ 2002; 324 (7350): 1350.

7 2003 Guide to the preparation, use and quality assurance of blood components, 9th Edition. Council of Europe Publishing.

8 James V, Hill J: National audit of new and lapsed donor deferrals. Transfusion Medicine 2002; 12 (Suppl): 50.

9 Farrell K, Ferguson E, James V, Lowe KC: Confidence in the safety of blood for transfusion: the effect of message framing. Transfusion 2002; 41 (11): 1335-1340

10 Calman KC: The language of risk: a question of trust. Transfusion 2001; 41 (11): 1326-1328.

11 Calman KC: Cancer: science and society and the communication of risk. BMJ 1996; 313 (7060): 799-802.

12 Lee DH, Paling JE, Blajchman MA: A new tool for communicating transfusion risk information. Transfusion 1998; 38 (2): 184-188.

13 Millennium Festival of Medicine: Transfusion Medicine 2001; 11: 119-145.

14 Soldan K, Sinka K: Evaluation of the de-selection of men, who have had sex with men, from blood donation in England. Vox Sang 2003 (in press).

15 Soldan K, Barbara JAJ, Ramsay ME, Hall AJ: Estimation of the risk of hepatitis B virus, hepatitis C virus and human immunodeficiency virus infectious donations entering the blood supply in England, 1993-2001. Vox Sang 2003 (in press).

Useful Web Sites

www.transfusionguidelines.org.uk
www.bcshguidelines.org
www.nice.org.uk
www.sign.ac.uk
www.agreecollaboration.org
www.guideline.gov/body_home. asp

Dr. V. James, National Blood Service, Sheffield Centre, Longley Lane, Sheffield, S5 7JN, United Kingdom.
E-mail: virge.james@nbs.nhs.uk

Vyas GN, Williams AE (eds): Advances in Transfusion Safety.
Dev Biol (Basel). Basel, Karger, 2005, vol 120, p 215.

SESSION XV

Panel and Open Discussion

Moderator: *M. Brecher*

Vyas GN, Williams AE (eds): Advances in Transfusion Safety.
Dev Biol (Basel). Basel, Karger, 2005, vol 120, pp 217-218.

What Drives Transfusion Practice?

Moderator: *M. Brecher*

Panelists: *M.F. Murphy, T.S. Kickler, M.H. Kanter, L.T. Goodnough*

Panel proceedings summarized by: *A.E. Williams*

Dr. Brecher posed three questions for the panel to consider:

1. *What drives change in transfusion practice?*
2. *How should proposed changes in transfusion practice be prioritized?*
3. *When should changes in transfusion practice be made mandatory?*

As demonstrated by published surveys of transfusion practice and retrospective assessments of transfusion use among homogeneous patient populations, there is evidence that much variation still exists in the degree of transfusion support in conjunction with medical and surgical procedures. While the universal goal is to obtain maximum therapeutic benefit for patients at the least cost and lowest risk, there are many differing opinions.

The panelists addressed the first discussion question in several different ways. The first was to indicate the factors which, rightly or wrongly, work to drive transfusion practice today. These include the recognized need for red cell support due to anaemia or haemorrhage, but also include physician responses to symptomatic cardiovascular response upon ambulation, such as syncope, tachycardia, or dyspnea. There appears to be a residual fear of under-transfusion in parts of the medical community that, when combined with poor physician understanding of transfusion benefits and risks, leads to unnecessary blood transfusion.

Other panelists chose to address the question in terms of the factors that **should** drive changes in transfusion practice. Among those discussed were adequate physician knowledge about risks and benefits, availability of credible transfusion benchmarks based upon well-designed multicentre trial data, and transfusion practice oversight that is appropriately targeted. It was argued that while numerous transfusion practice guidelines have been developed and made available to the blood transfusion community, they have not been offered in such a way that they draw widespread physician attention and adherence. While several panel representatives argued that science was the primary driving force in establishing practice guidelines at their institutions, others maintained that the most effective vehicles for change are focused media and legal attention at a peer institution. One panelist suggested that lessons should be taken from the pharmaceutical industry, which appears to have developed highly targeted measures to influence physicians with respect to prescription practices.

Randomized multicentre trials of patient outcome in response to different haemoglobin target levels; e.g. the TRICC Study, were discussed as being exceedingly valuable, but potentially flawed by substantial selection biases. These biases were explained as potentially arising from the fact that physician agreement was necessary before random selection of patients. Given that the best interests of the patient were the principal concern of the treating physician, the physician would be likely to approve random assignment to a liberal or restricted transfusion arm when it was pre-assessed that the patient could tolerate either treatment.

The actual process of making and communicating transfusion policy decisions at the local level was discussed extensively. Social networks among doctors need to be recognized, including those that involve different medical specialities. It should also be recognized that there are likely to be opinion-leaders among the stakeholder physicians. Support from such opinion-leaders can be critical to successful change. Local stakeholders, from both the medical and patient community, need to be identified and involved. Educated patients frequently wish to be closely involved with their medical care. Examples were given from large institutions where the extensive solicitation of ideas and attitudes from hospital user-group communities helped to support policies of reduced transfusions, increased use of haemodilution, and optimized use of growth factors. In one facility, such interaction even led to the development of a bloodless medicine programme.

In the area of local policy development, it was agreed there should be a transparent conceptual framework under which decisions will be made, including which transfusion-related measures are and are not potential targets for standardization. These decisions then need to rest on a sound medical, operational, legal and financial footing.

And once decisions for change are made, policy-makers need to make sure that implementation of mandated changes does not disrupt delivery of services and patient care.

A frequent hurdle to successful long-term change is an absence of "observability" i.e., knowing whether a relative advantage was actually derived from a particular change. Observability may be particularly important when changing from a familiar to an unknown practice. A pilot study approach with defined outcome measures may help to determine not only the value, but also the unexpected pitfalls of more comprehensive change.

List of Participants

ADEL SEDKY Hebatallah, Lab Top Labs, 29 Shehab Street, Mohandessin, Cairo, Egypt.

AKOLKAR Pradip, CBER/FDA, 1401 Rockville Pike, HFM-310, Rockville, MD 20852, USA.

ALEXANDER Samantha, AABB, 8101 Glenbrook Rd, Bethesda, MD 20814-2747, USA.

ALFORD Bernadette, Vi technologies, 134 Coolidge Ave, Watertown, MA 02472-2815, USA.

ALLAIN Jean-Pierre, University of Cambridge, Long Road, Cambridge CB2 2PT, United Kingdom.

ALMS Linda, MGA, FDA, OBRR, DBA, 1401 Rockville Pike, HFM-375 Woc 1, Rockville, MD 20852, USA.

ALTER Harvey, Dept. of Transfusion Med., Clinical Center, MSC 1184, NIH 9000 Rockville Pike, Bethesda, MD 20892, USA.

ALVING Barbara, National Heart, Lung & Blood, 31 Center Dr., Bldg 31 M5A47, Bethesda, MD 20892, USA.

AMENDT Linda, OBRR, Center for Biologics Eval., 1401 Rockville Pike, HFM-300, Rockville, MD 20852-1448, USA.

ASHER David, Lab. of Bacterial and Parasitic Agents, FDA/CBER/DETTD, NLRC RMB128, HFM-313, 1401 Rockville Pike, Rockville, MD 20852-1448, USA.

AYOB Yasmin, National Blood Centre, Jalan Tun Razak, 50400 Kuala Lumpur, Malaysia.

BAEZA Federico, Baxter Transfusion Therapies, Parque Empresarial San Fernando, Edificio Londres, ES-28830 Madrid, Spain.

BALLAS Samir, Thomas Jefferson University, 1015 Walnut St., Cardeza Foundation, Philadelphia, PA 19107-5005, USA.

BARR John, V J Technologies Inc., 134 Coolidge Ave, Watertnon, MA 02472, USA.

BENJAMIN Richard, American Red Cross, 180 Rustcraft Rd, Ste 115, Dedham, MA 02026-4594, USA.

BHARUCHA Zarin, Bombay Red Cross Blood Centre, Town Hall Compound, Shahid Bhagat Singh Rd, Mumbai – 400001, India.

BIANCO Celso, America's Blood Center, 725 15th Street, Washington, DC 2005, USA.

BISWAS Robin, FDA/CBER, 1401 Rockville Pike, HFM-310, Ste 200, Rockville, MD 20852, USA.

BLAJCHMAN Morris, Pathology Department, McMaster University, 1200 Main St. W., HSC-2N34, Hamilton, Ont., Canada L8N3Z5.

BLUM Karan, FDA/Center for Biologics Eval., 1401 Rockville Pike, Rockville, MD 20852, USA.

BRECHER, Mark, UNC Dept of Pathology, UNC Hospitals, Campus Box 7525, 101 Manning Dr., Chapel Hill, NC 27599-7525, USA.

BRITTENHAM Gary, Columbia University, Harkness Pavillon, Rm HP568, 630 West, 18th Street, New York, NY 100032, USA.

BROWN Paul, 7815 Exeter Road, Bethesda, MD 20814, USA.

BULT Jan, Plasma Protein Therapeutics Assoc., 147 Old Solomons Island Rd, Annapolis, MD 21401, USA.

BUNKENS Helena, Gambro Bct, 10811 West Collins Ave, Lakewood, CO 80215, USA.

BUSCH Michael, Blood Systems Research Institute, 270 Masonic Ave., San Francisco, CA 94904, USA.

CALLAGHAN Elizabeth, FDA, 1401 Rockville Pike, HFM-370, Rockville, MD 20852, USA.

CALMANN Mark, Ortho-Clinical Diagnostics, 1001 US Highway 202, Raritan, NJ 08869-1424, USA.

CARR-GREER Allene, AABB, 8101 Glenbrook Rd, Bethesda, MD 20814-2747, USA.

CARSON Jeffrey, Robert Wood Johnson Univ Hosp., 125, Paterson Street, Suite 5100, New Brunswick, NJ 08903-0019, USA.

CHAMBERS Linda, Biomedical Headquarters, American Red Cross, 2025 E. St. NW, Washington, D.C. 20006, USA.

CHANG Andrew, CBER FDA, 1401 Rockville Pike, HFM-330, Rockville, MD 20852, USA.

CHAPMAN John, Vitex, 134 Coolidge Ave, Watertown, MA 02472-2815, USA.

CHAPMAN Paul, Roche Molecular Systems, 4300 Hacienda Dr., Pleasanton, CA 94588-2722, USA.

CIARALDI Judy, FDA, 1401 Rockville Pike, Rockville, MD 20852-3524, USA.

CLARK Kenneth, Intern. Transfusion Team, CDC, 1600 Clifton Rd, NE, Atlanta, GA 30329-4027, USA.

CLIBOURN Douglas, Zymequest Inc, 100 Cummings Ctr, Ste 436th, Beverly, MA 01915-6122, USA.

COCROFT Cara, Baxter Healthcare, 1627 Lake Cook Road, LCIV-2 N, Deerfield, Il 60015, USA.

CONLAN Maureen, Cerus Corporation, 2411 Stanwell Drive, Concord, CA 94519, USA.

CONLEY Gilliam, FDA/CBER/OBRR, Div. of Blood, 1401 Rockville Pike, HFM-375, Rockville, MD 20852, USA.

CORBIN Frank, Navigant Biotechnologies, 10811 W Collins Ave., Lakewood, CO 80215, USA.

COUNTS Frank, 11804 Sycamore Rd, Mount Vernon, OH 43050-8543, USA.

COWAN Elliot, FDA/CBER/OBRR/DETTD, 1401 Rockville Pike, HFM-310, Rockville, MD 20852, USA.

CRUZ Jose R. Pan American Health Organization, 525 23[Rd] Street, NW, Washington, DC 20037, USA.

CUMMING Paul, Talisman Ltd., 1740 Burning Tree Drive, Vienna, VA 22182, USA.

DARIOTIS Jeanne, CEO, Community Blood Center, 1731 Riggins Rd, Tallahassee, Fl 32308-5317, USA.

DAVIS Guanah D., Process Design American Red Cross, 1616 Fort Myer Dr., 15th Floor, Arlington, VA 22209-3100, USA.

DAVIS Joyce, Medical Marketing Consultants, 13228 Executive Park Terrace, Germantown, MD 20874, USA.

DE NATRIS Theo, Biomerieux Boseind 15, PO Box 23, NL-5280 AA Boxtel, The Netherlands.

DELVALLE Carlos, NY Blood Center, 310 E 67th St., New York, NY 10021-6273, USA.

DHINGRA Neelam, Transfusion Safety Unit, World Health Organization, CH-1211 Geneva 27, Switzerland.

DIAMOND Richard, FDA/CBER NIH Bldg. 29b, Room 326, Rockville, MD 20852, USA.

DODD Roger, American Red Cross Blood, Jerome H. Holland Lab., 15601 Crabbs Branch Way, Rockville, MD 20855, USA.

DUPUIS Kent, Cerus Corporation, 2411 Stanwell Drive, Concord, CA 94520, USA.

ELFATH Dean, Baxter Healthcare Corp., Rt 120 and Wilson Road, Round Lake, Il 60073, USA.

ENGLISH Kieran, Chiron Corporation, 4560 Horton St., MS Z-300, Emeryville, CA 94608, USA.

EPSTEIN Jay, FDA/CBER/OBRR, HFM-300, 1401 Rockville Pike, Rockville, MD 20852-1448, USA.

EVERS Theo, Euro Plasma Fractionation, Plesmanlaan 125, Postbus 9190, NL-1060 CX Amsterdam, The Netherlands.

FANG Chyang, American Red Cross, 15601 Crabbs Branch Way, Rockville, MD 20855-2743, USA.

FARRUGIA Albert, Blood & Tissue Unit, Office of Devices, Australian TGA, P.O. Box 100, Woden, ACT 2606, Australia.

FARSHID Mahmood, FDA/CBER/DH, 1401 Rockville Pike, HFM-345, NIH Bldg.29, Rockville, MD 20852, USA.

FAYAD Sawson, C/o Lab Top Labs, 29 Shehab Street, Mohandessin Cairo, Cairo, Egypt.

FIPPS Donald R., Blood & Plasma, American Red Cross, 1616 Fort Myer Dr., 15th Floor, Arlington, VA 22209-3100, USA.

FITZPATRICK Mike, America's Blood Centers, 725 15th St., NW, Ste 700, Washington, DC 20005, USA.

FOSS Mary, Division of Transf. Medicine, Mayo Clinic Rochester, 200 First Street, SW, Hilton 253, Rochester, MN 55905-0002, USA.

FRANCIS Kori, FDA/CBER/OBRR/DETTD, 1401 Rockville Pike, Ste 200, HFM-323, Rockville, MD 20852, USA.

FRENETTE Donna, Roche Molecular Systems, 4300 Hacienda Dr., Pleasanton, CA 94588-2722, USA.

FRIEDMAN Len, Terumo Medical Corporation, 2101 Cottontail Lane, Somerset, NJ 08873, USA.

GALLARDA James, Roche Molecular Systems, 4300 Hacienda Dr., Pleasanton, CA 94588-2722, USA.

GAO Guang, CBER, 1401 Rockville Pike, HFM-310, Rockville, MD 20852, USA.

GARCIA Marcela, Pan American Health Organization, 525 23rd Street, NW, Washington, DC 20037, USA.

GASTINEAU Dennis, Mayo Clinic, 200 1st St. SW, Rochester, MN 55905-0002, USA.

GAWRYL Maria, Biopure Corporation, 11 Hurley Street, Cambridge, MA 02141, USA.

GHOSH Suanta, New Zealand Blood Service, Waikato, Hamilton, New Zealand.

GILCHER Ron, Oklahoma Blood Institute, 1001 N. Lincoln Blvd., Oklahoma City, OK 73104-3299, USA.

GILL Jennifer, American Red Cross,15601 Crabbs Branch Way, Rockville, MD 20855-2736, USA.

GILSTAD Colleen, Armed Services, Blood Bank Center, 8901 Wisconsin Avenue, Bethesda, MD 20889-5600, USA.

GLYNN Simone, Health Studies, Westat, 1650 Research Blvd, Room WB280, Rockville, MD 20850, USA.

GOLDING Basil, DH/CBER/FDA, 1401 Woodmont, Rockville, MD 20852, USA.

GOODMAN Rick, Ortho-Clinical Diagnostics, 1001 US Highway 202, Raritan, NJ 08869-1424, USA.

GOODNOUGH Tim, Stanford University Medical Center, Transfusion Service, 300 Pasteur Drive, Rm H1402, M/C 5626, Stanford, CA 94305-5626, USA.

GRAY Joyce, AABB, 8101 Glenbrook Rd, Bethesda, MD 20814-2747, USA.

GREGORY Kay, Regulatory Affairs, AABB, 8101 Glenbrook Rd, Bethesda, MD 20814-2747, USA.

GROENER Albrecht, Aventis Behring GmbH, PO Box 1230, DE-35002 Marburg, Germany.

GUST Ian, University of Melbourne, Gratton St., Parkville, Melbourne 3010, Australia.

HARDIMAN Anthony, Ortho-Clincal Diagnostics, 1001 US Highway 202, Raritan, NJ 08869-1424, USA.

HARLEY Patricia, FDA, 1401 Rockville Pike, Room 400 S, Rockville, MD 20852-1428, USA.

HARVATH Liana, Division of Blood National Hear, Lung & Blood, 6701 Rockledge Dr., Bethesda, MD 20892, USA.

HASEBE Hiroaki (Harry), 201 Great Valley Parkway, Malvern, PA 19355, USA.

HASSAN Salwa M., C/o Lab Top Labs, 29 Shehab Street, Mohandessin Cairo, Cairo, Egypt.

HAWARDEN Vick, AABB, 8101 Glenbrook Rd, Bethesda, MD 20814-2747, USA.

HEDGES Teresa, Cerug Corporation, 2411 Stanwell Drive, Concord, CA 94520, USA.

HERRON Ross, American Red Cross, 1130 South Vermont Ave, Los Angeles, CA 90006, USA.

HESS John, Blood Bank, N2W 50A, Baltimore, MD 20817, USA.

HEWLETT Indira, CBER/FDA, 9000 Wisconsin Ave, Bethesda, MD 20892 USA.

HEYNS Anton S., S. African Blood Transfusion Service, Private Bag X14, Weltereden Park 1715, South Africa.

HOUTCHENS Robert, Process Development Biopure Corp., 11 Hurley St., Cambridge, MA 02141, USA.

HROVAT Teresa, American Red Cross, 1616 Fort Myer Dr, Rm 1515, Arlington, VA 22209-3100, USA.

HULVEY Robyn, AABB, 8101 Glenbrook Rd, Bethesda, MD 20814-2747, USA.

ISHIMOTO Janet, FDA, 1401 Rockville Pike, Rockville, MD 20852-3524, USA.

JACOBS Mary Beth, US Food and Drug Administration, 1401 Rockville Pike, HFM-400, Rockville, MD 20852, USA.

JAMES Virge, National Blood Service, Sheffield Centre, Longley Lane, Sheffield, S5 7JN, United Kingdom.

JONES Liz, American Red Cross, 1616 Fort Myer Dr. 15th Floor, Arlington, VA 22209-3100, USA.

KANTER Michael, 393 E., Walnut Street, Pasadena, CA 91188, USA.

KAPLAN Hal, Dept of Pathology, Columbia University, 622 West, 168th Street, New York, NY 10032, USA.

KELLEY Diane, U.S. Food and Drug Administration, 1350 Piccard Dr., Rockville, MD 20850-4307, USA.

KICKLER Tom, Johns Hopkins Hospital, School of Medicine, Weinberg Bldg, Rm 2333, 401 N Broadway Street, Baltimore, MD 21231, USA.

KLEIN Harvey, Dept of Transfusion Medicine, NIH, Warren G. Magnuson Clinical Center, Bldg 10, Rm IC-711, Bethesda, MD 20892, USA.

KLEINMAN Steve, 1281 Rockcrest Avenue, Victoria, BC V9A-4W4, Canada.

KO Hon Som, Food and Drug Administration, 1404 Rockville Pike, HFM-392, Rockville, MD 20852, USA.

KOISTINEN Jukka, FRC Blood Transfusion Service, Kivihaantie 7, FI-00310 Helsinki, Finland.

KOLINS Jerry, American Red Cross Blood, 7675 Mesa College Drive, San Diego, CA 92111-5341, USA.

KOSANKE Joanne, 995 E Broad St., Columbus, OH 43205-1322, USA.

KRETSCHMER Volker, Institute of Transf. Med. & Haemost., University Hospital, Conradistrasse, DE-35033, Marburg, Germany.

KURAMOTO I. Ken, Chiron Corporation, 4560 Horton St, MS Z-300, Emeryville, CA 94608, USA.

LASSEN Ursula, DRK-BTS-NSTOB, Eldagsener Str. 38, DE-31832 Springe, Germany.

LAWRENCE Teri, Ortho-Cinical Diagnostics, 1001 US Highway, 202, Raritan, NJ 08869-1424, USA.

LE GEAR Michele, Ortho-Clinical Diagnostics, 1001 US Highway, 202, Raritan, NJ 08869-1424, USA.

LEIBY David, Transmissible Dis. Dept., Jerome H. Holland Lab., American Red Cross, 15601 Crabbs Branch Way, Rockville, MD 20855, USA.

LELKENS Charles, Ministry of Defense, Plesmanlaan 1c, NL-2333 BZ Leiden, The Netherlands.

LEPARC German, Florida Blood Services, 10100 9th. Street, North St., Petersburg, Fl 33716, USA.

LESLEY Peter, Ottawa Center, 85 Plymouth Street, Ottawa, Ont 5I5 3E2, Canada.

LEWIS Richard, 39275 Snow Lane, Lorettsville, VA 20180, USA.

LODER Natasha, The Economist, 25 St., James Street, London, SW1A 1HG, United Kingdom.

LOEWER Johannes, Paul-Erlich-Institute, Paul-Ehrlich-Str. 51-59, DE-63225 Langen, Germany.

LOFTUS Patrick, Canadian Blood Services, 4750 Oak Street, Vancouver, BC V6E 1L9, Canada.

LONG Karen, Roche, 4300 Hacrenda Drive, Pleasanton, CA 94588, USA.

LONSER Roland, Hinsdale Hospital Blood Bank, 120 E Oak St., Hinsdale, Il 60521-3829, USA.

LOPEZ-PLAZA Ileana, Univ of Pittsburg, 1434 Towne Square Dr., Allison Park, PA 15101, USA.

LOZIER Jay, FDA/CBER/OBRR/DH/LH, 1404 Rockville Pike, HFM-340, Rockville, MD 20852, USA.

MACLEARY Debbie, Riddle Memorial Hospital, 1068 W Baltimore Pike, Medin, PA 19063, USA.

MATHEWS Michael, Hemosol, 8 Woodhollow Rd, Ste 301, Parsippany, NJ 07054-2829, USA.

McCOMBIE Nancy, Health Canada, Tunney's Pasture Bldg. #6, Al0601E2, Ottawa, Ont. K2E 7V4, Canada.

McCURDY Paul, Paul R. McCurdy, 6452 Elmdale Rd, Alexandria, VA 22312-1317, USA.

McDONOUGH Brian, Ortho Clinical Diagnositcs, 1001 US Highway 202, Raritan, NJ 08869-1424, USA.

McKINNEY Carlene, AABB, 8101 Glenbrook Rd, Bethesda, MD 20814-2747, USA.

MELMED Russell, American Red Cross, 5601 Crabbs Branch Way, Rockville, MD 20855-2736, USA.

MENY Geraldyn, American Red Cross, 700 Spring Garden St., Penn-Jersey Region, Philadelphia, PA 19123-3594, USA.

MIED Paul, FDA/CBER, 1400 Rockville Pike, HFM-310, Rockville, MD 20852, USA.

MIKKELSON Niels, IFBDO, Danish Blood Donor Assoc., Vesterbrogade 191, DK-1800 Frederiksberg, Denmark.

MILLER Reed, The Gray Sheet - FDC Reports, Inc., 5550 Friendship Blvd., Suite One, Chevy Chase, MD 20815, USA.

MILLER William V, 330 W Madison Ave, Saint Louis, MO 63122-4105, USA.

MING Zhu Yong, Shanghai (Red Cross) Blood Center, #1191, Hong Qiao Rd., Shanghai 200051, China.

MOORE S. Breanndon, Mayo Clinic, 200 1st St. SW, Rochester, MN 55905-0002, USA.

MURPHY Mike, Nat. Blood Service, Dept of Haematol., John Radcliffe Hospital, The University Oxford, Oxford 0X3 9BQ, United Kingdom.

NAKHASI Hira, DETTD/OBRR/CBER/FDA, 8800 Rockville Pike Bldg. 29, Rm 222, Bethesda, MD 20892, USA.

NEERAARD Lauran, The Associated Press, 2021 K Street, NW, Suite 600, Washington, DC 20006, USA.

NELSON Kenrad, USDA, Johns Hopkins Univ. School of Hygiene, 615 N. Wolfe, Rm. E-7132, Baltimore, MD 21205, USA.

NEMO George, Transfusion Medicine & Cell, 6701 Rockledge Dr., Bethesda, MD 20892, USA.

NIGHTINGALE Stephen, Burntside Partners, Inc., 4703 Broad Brook Dr., Bethesda, MD 20814-3903, USA.

NIU Manette, FDA/CBER/OBRR/DBA, 1401 Rockville Pike, HFM-370, Rockville, MD 20852, USA.

ORTON Sharyn, CBER, OBRR, Division of Blood Application, FDA, 1401 Rockville Pike, Rockville, MD 20852, USA.

OTTER Jean, AABB, 8101 Glenbrook Rd, Bethesda, MD 20814-2747, USA.

PEOPLES Barbara, American Red Cross, 2025 East Street, NW, Washington, DC 20006, USA.

PEREZ-ROSALES Maria D., Pan American Health Organization, 525 23 Rd Street, NW, Washington, DC 20037, USA.

PHELPS Bruce, Chiron Corporation, 4560 Horton Street, MS Z-300, Emeryville, CA 94608, USA.

PICCARDO Pedro, CBER, 1404 Rockville Pike, HFM 310, Rockville, MD 20852, USA.

PINKERTON Peter, Sunnybrook & Women's Col HSC, Room B 204, 2075 Bayview Ave, Toronto, Ont M4N 3M5, Canada.

PINOVER Kathy, Bonfils Blood Center, 717 Yosemite Street, Denver, CO 80230, USA.

POINDEXTER Betsy, FDA/CBER, 1401 Rockville Pike, HFM-335, Rockville, MD 20852, USA.

POSTERNAK Barry, Kensico Capital, 200 Park Avenue, New York, NY 10166, USA.

PRATT Kasie, American Red Cross, 15601 Crabbs Branch Way, Rockville, MD 20855-2736, USA.

RAZZAQUE Abdur, Office of Blood Research, 1401 Rockville Pike, HFM-394, Rockville, MD 20852, USA.

REILLY Patricia, Terumo Medical Corporation, 2101 Cottontail Lane, Somerset, NJ 08873, USA.

RICHARDS Karen, Chiron Corporation, 4560 Horton St., Mailstop N1-118, Emeryville, CA 94608-2900, USA.

RUDMANN Sally, The Ohio State University, School of Allied Med. Professions, Div. of Med. Technology, Atwell Hall, 453 West 10th Ave., Columbus, OH 43210, USA.

RUTA Martin, FDA, 1401 Rockville Pike, Rockville, MD 20852, USA.

SALATA Jeanne, W Reed Army Inst of Research, 503 Robert Grant Ave, Rm 1N56, Silver Spring, MD 20910-7500, USA.

SANDLER S. Gerald, Dept of Lab. Medicine, Georgetown Univ. Hospital, 3800 Reservoir Rd, NW, Washington, DC 20007, USA.

SAZAMA Kathleen, The University of Texas, Anderson Cancer Center, 1515 Holcombe Blvd, Unit 800, Houston, TX 77030, USA.

SCHIFFER Charles, Div. of Hematology/Oncology, Karmanos Cancer Institute, HWCRC – 4th Floor, 4100 John R., Detroit, MI 48302, USA.

SCHREIBER George, Health Studies, Westat, 1650 Research Blvd, Rockville, MD 20850, USA.

SCOTT Dot, OBRR/CBER/FDA, 8800 Rockville Pike, Bethesda, MD 20892, USA.

SEITZ Rainer, Paul-Ehrlich-Institute, Paul-Ehrlich-Str. 51-59, DE-63225 Langen, Germany.

SESAN Adeyemi, Engineering Compuscope, 3 Oluwa Lane off Olokodana St. Eb/Meta, Lagos 23401, Nigeria.

SHAN Hua, Johns Hopkins Hospital, 10272 Breconshire Rd, Ellicott City, MD 21042-5854, USA.

SHER Graham, Canadian Blood Services, 1800 Alta Vista Drive, Ottawa, Ont. K1G 4J5, Canada.

SIBINGA SMIT Cees, IDTM and SCS, P.O. Box 11085, NL-9700 CB Groningen, The Netherlands.

SICKLER Van, American Red Cross, 2025 East Street, NW, Washington, DC 20006, USA.

SIMAK Jan, FDA/CBER NIH, Bldg. 29b, Room 326, Rockville, MD 20852, USA.

SIMNICEANU Alexandria, Al 0201c1 Finance Building, Tuneys Pasture, Ottawa, Ont K1A 1B9, Canada.

SIMON Toby, Tricore Reference Lab, 1001 Woodward Pl., NE, Albuquerque, NM 87102, USA.

SINK Bonnie, Natl. Institutes of Health, 10 Center Drive, MSC1184, Bldg. 10, Rm. 1c711, Bethesda MD 20892-0001, USA.

SMALLWOOD Linda, CBER/FDA, 1401 Rockville Pike, HFM-302, Rockville, MD 20782, USA.

SNYDER Ed, Yale University School of Medicine, 333 Cedar Street, New Aven, CT 06510, USA.

STACK Gary, VA Connecticut Healthcare System, 950 Campbell Avenue, West Haven, CT 06516, USA.

STRENGERS Paul, Intl Soc. Blood Transfusions, Plesmanstraat 125, NL-1006 AX Amsterdam, The Netherlands.

SWEENEY John P. Miles and Stockbridge, 10 Light Street, Baltimore, MD 21202, USA.

SYLVESTER Ruth, Armed Services Blood Program, 5109 Leesburg Pike, Room 698, Falls Church, VA 22041-3258, USA.

TABOR Ed, Office of Blood Research, 1401 Rockville Pike, HFM-300, Rockville, MD 20852, USA.

TAFF Rolf, Office of Blood Research, 1401 Rockville Pike, HFM-313, Rockville, MD 20852, USA.

TERRY Beverly, 12958 Elgin Drive, Denver, CO 80239-4419, USA.

THIAGARAJAN Perumal, Baylor College of Medicine, 2002 Holcome Blvd, Vamc mail # 113, Houston, TX 77030, USA.

TILLSON Elizabeth, Regulatory Affairs & Quality, Cerus Corporation, 2411 Stanwell Dr., Concord, CA 94520-4810, USA.

ULZ Laura, Seattle Cancer Care Alliance, 825 Eastland Ave, E LA- 210, Seattle, WA 98109, USA.

UPCRAFT Gerald, University California, Davis, 514 Flicker Ave, Davis, CA 95616-0178, USA.

VAN der POEL Cees, Sanquin Blood Supply Found, Plesmanlaan 125, NL-1066 CX Amsterdam, The Netherlands.

VASILYEVA Irina, American Red Cross, 15601 Crabbs Branch Way, Rockville, MD 20855, USA.

VAUGHN James, Cerus Corporation, 2411 Stanwell Drive, Concord, CA 94520, USA.

VINELLI Elizabeth, Cruz Roja Hondurena, Programa Nacional De Sangre, 2 Avenida de Comayaguela, M.D.C. Honduras.

VOSTAL Jaroslav, Laboratory of Cellular Hemat, 8800 Rockville Pike, Rockville, MD 20892, USA.

VYAS Girish, Univ. of CA, School of Medicine, 513 Parnassus Ave., Rm S-561, San Francisco, CA 94143-0100, USA.

WALLER Charles, PPTA Europe, 114/5 Blvd Brand Whitlock, BE-1200 Brussels, Belgium.

WEBB Marlon, American Red Cross Biomedical Services, 2025 E. St. NW (5th floor NE 5040C), Washington, D.C. 20006, USA.

WEI Thomas, 405 Lexington Ave, Fl. 58th Chrysler Center. New York. NY 10174-0002. USA.

WHITAKER Barbee, Alta Chem. Pharma Ltd., 9411 20 Ave., Edmonton, Alberta, Canada, T6N 1E5.

WILCZEK Joe, FDA/CBER, 1401 Rockville Pike, HFM-302, Rockville, MD 20852, USA.

WILL Robert, Natl CJD Surveillance Unit, Dept of Neurosciences, Western General Hospital, Crewe Rd, Edinburgh EH4 2XU, United Kingdom.

WILLIAMS Alan, OBRR/CBER/FDA, 1401 Rockville Pike, HFM-370, Rockville, MD 20852, USA.

WILLKOMMEN Hannelore, Clearant Inc, 401 Professional Drive, Gaithersburg, MD 20879, USA.

WILSON Janine, 310 E 67th Street, New York, NY 10021, USA.

WONG Lynn, American Red Cross, 15601 Crabbs Branch Way, Rockville, MD 20855, USA.

WORTHAM Samuel T., Medical Group Pall Corporation, 2200 Northern Blvd., East Hills, NY 11548, USA.

YU Mei-ying (Monica), Divison of Hematology, 1401 Rockville Pike, HGM-345, Rockville, MD 20852, USA.

ZENMANN Kenneth, FDA/CBER, 14800 Soft Wind Dr., North Potomac, MD 20878, USA.

ZOU Shimian, American Red Cross, 15601 Crabbs Branch Way, Rockville, MD 20855, USA.